To my children Paul and Kathryn and grandsons Scott, Dylan and Kieran, who all taught me an awful lot about babies!

Acknowledgements

I'd like to thank Claire Plimmer for commissioning this book and casting a 'mum's eye' over the content. I'm also very grateful to Denyse Kirkby, midwifery lecturer and author of My *Mini Midwife*, and Sally Lewis, author and expert in antenatal and postnatal health and fitness, for taking time out of their busy schedules to write the forewords. Thanks also to Debbie Chapman and Sandy Draper for their very helpful editorial input.

Disclaimer

Every effort has been made to ensure that the information in this book is accurate and current at the time of publication. The author and the publisher cannot accept responsibility for any misuse or misunderstanding of any information contained herein, or any loss, damage or injury, be it health, financial or otherwise, suffered by any individual or group acting upon or relying on information contained herein. None of the opinions or suggestions in this book is intended to replace medical opinion. If you have concerns about your, or your baby's health, please seek professional advice.

CONTENTS

AUTHOR'S NOTE

Although it's a number of years since I had my two children, my experiences of being a grandparent and of researching and writing this book made me realise that nothing has really changed: new parents face exactly the same concerns and issues that my then husband and I did.

The first three months were the most demanding; everything was new to us, I'd never even changed a baby's nappy, let alone bathed a baby. Once I had left hospital there was no support with breastfeeding and no one talked about how difficult it is having a new baby. For those first few weeks, life seemed to revolve around breastfeeds and nappy changes – my then husband soon realised that if he wanted to eat, he would have to cook!

It wasn't any easier the second time around, as by then I had a 14-month old toddler, as well as a new baby to cope with. On the day my husband returned to work after a week's leave, I was still in my dressing gown at 1 p.m. and my son had spent most of the morning in his high chair, while I breastfed his baby sister. I remember wondering how on earth I would ever manage to take a bath or go shopping. On top of all that, my daughter developed colic when she was a couple of weeks old, so I had to deal with her crying for long periods. Then, of course, there was the broken sleep due to the night feeds. But I quickly learned how to juggle caring for two babies and as time went on I started to relax and enjoy being a mother.

The truth is the reality of having a baby is much different to how we think it's going to be. Nothing can prepare you for it, but I hope that this book will give you some insight into what to expect in the first three months of your baby's life and help you cope with the worries and issues you may encounter – including lack of sleep, lack of time and feeling overwhelmed at times – safe in the knowledge that you most definitely are not alone. Despite the challenges, at the end of the first three months, I'm sure you'll agree that becoming a parent is one of the best things you ever did!

FOREWORD

from Denyse Kirkby – registered midwife (NMC), registered midwifery teacher (NMC), registered public health practitioner (UKPHPR) and author of *My Mini Midwife*

The very best parenting is often discovered through perseverance and a willingness to try out new techniques, rather than through prior expertise or specialised training. However, when new parents are suffering from sleep deprivation and a desire to only give their baby the very best of their care, it is a challenge to be able to think of new ways to satisfy their baby's demands.

The New Parents' Survival Guide offers parents a variety of techniques to try, with anecdotes from other parents as well as the author's own experiences with parenting, and the reasoning behind her advice.

No new experience is the same for every parent, but this little book is crammed full of suggestions and there is bound to be something in here that will support every parent with deciphering their baby's needs, and with getting themselves as prepared as possible beforehand.

The honest, insightful and detailed sections on the highs and lows of parenting in the early months turns *The New Parents' Survival Guide* into a map that will show parents how to get to the other side of the fourth trimester with their sense of humour intact.

FOREWORD
from Sally Lewis – ante and post natal health advisor

No one ever said being a parent was easy. During the many years I have spent teaching on both ante and post natal classes I have heard plenty of advice offered to new prospective parents. From family members, to friends, even complete strangers, everyone it appears has an opinion and many, as you will probably discover, are best ignored. But home alone, the prospects of caring for, and understanding your newborn baby's needs and requirements in those first few months can feel daunting, and at times overwhelming. That's where this book provides the perfect companion. With its easy-to-read style the book allows you to dip in and out of the sections you need as you negotiate your way through the early days of parenthood.

The New Parents' Survival Guide offers practical, simple advice; indeed it's a bit like having a very reassuring mother or best friend sitting beside you offering help and support as you begin your journey into parenthood, without them having to actually move in.

INTRODUCTION

Having a baby is an amazing, joyful experience, but it brings with it a new set of responsibilities that can feel overwhelming at times – especially in the first three months. While there is a wealth of information out there on how to care for your new baby, much of it glosses over the reality of life as a first-time parent.

This book aims to offer a more realistic picture of what caring for a newborn is like, so it contains real-life new parents' experiences and tips, and offers advice on the issues you are most likely to encounter, such as feeding and sleeping problems, tiredness, how to cope if your baby cries a lot and, just as importantly, how to look after yourself – especially in the early days when you are feeling exhausted from the massive physical and emotional upheaval you have just undergone. While most parents experience similar problems, what is clear from the real-life stories is that there is no one 'right' way to care for your baby, as they are all individuals and *you* are the expert on your own baby and what is best for you both.

In this book you will find chapters on what to buy in preparation for your baby's arrival, basic baby care and first-aid skills, both for emergencies and treating minor ailments, such as nappy rash and colic. There's also information on how breastfeeding works, which will help you to understand the advice on how to breastfeed and how to overcome common problems. The book also looks at the pros and cons of breastfeeding, bottle-feeding and combination feeding to help you choose the method that best suits you and your baby.

You will also find out how to calm your crying baby, as well as how to settle them to sleep and establish a good sleep routine. All parents want to make sure that their baby is developing normally, so there is a chapter about the milestones your baby should reach in the first three months. The final chapter is all about you – the changes you are likely to notice in your body post-pregnancy, as well as how to look after yourself to enable you to cope with the physical and emotional demands of caring for your new baby. At the end of the book you will find details of useful products and helpful books and organisations. I hope you will find this book a helpful and reassuring resource as you begin your journey into parenthood.

CHAPTER 1
BE PREPARED

In the months before the birth you will naturally want to prepare for your baby's arrival. It makes sense to buy all of the equipment you will need at least a couple of months before your due date – just in case your baby decides to make their entrance earlier than expected! With so many baby products out there, it can be difficult to decide what you really need and what is just an optional extra, so this chapter offers a checklist of the essentials you will need in the first three months, as well as one or two items that could make life easier, but are not absolutely necessary. The suggested quantities are just a guide.

In this chapter:

▶ Prepare the nursery
▶ Designate some 'baby areas'

Checklist – have you got everything you need?

▶ Clothing
▶ Nappy changing
▶ Breastfeeding equipment
▶ Bottle-feeding equipment
▶ Bathing
▶ Sleeping
▶ Transport
▶ Useful extras
▶ Basic baby's first aid kit

Prepare the nursery

You might want to decorate the room that will eventually be your baby's nursery, even though your baby will be sleeping in your bedroom until they are at least six months; this is the current recommendation for safer sleeping – but you should not share a bedroom if you or your partner smokes. It is certainly a good idea to decorate the nursery before your baby is born, as it will be a lot harder to find the time when you have a new baby to care for. Also it's best to allow plenty of time for the nursery to air after painting or redecorating to avoid any strong fumes in the room when you start using it for your baby. The nursery will also be an ideal place to store a lot of their equipment and clothing.

Top tips on preparing your baby's nursery

▶ If you have more than one room to choose from, pick the one that is closest to your bedroom.

▶ Preferably it should be a quiet room away from noisy roads and places where children play.

▶ Choose plain, neutral colours such as cream or beige so that it will be easy to update the room with colourful murals or wall stickers, posters and bedding, as your child grows.

▶ Use low-fume or child-friendly paints and natural floor coverings, such as a wool carpet or wood flooring to reduce the number of chemicals your baby will be exposed to.

▶ Choose washable paint so it is easy to clean.

- ► Blackout blinds and heavy curtains will help to ensure your baby sleeps soundly.

- ► Choose cordless blinds to avoid the risk of entanglement.

- ► Don't put your baby's cot near a window or a radiator.

- ► A comfortable chair/rocking chair where you can cuddle your baby and perhaps share a bedtime song or story is a useful addition.

Designate some 'baby areas'

Think about where you will keep your baby's pram or buggy when it's not in use. Most people use the hall or a spot under the stairs, but if space is at a premium you could keep it in your car boot or in a secure shed or garage.

Designate an area in your living room where you can store your baby's nappies, toiletries and a few items of clothing, so that you always have them close to hand. A portable baby box or a baby-changing bag is ideal for keeping your baby's everyday essential items all in one place.

Checklist – have you got everything you need?

While it is important to make sure you have all of the necessary items you and your baby will need in the first few months, you don't need to go overboard. One new mum, Pam, pointed out that many of the things she bought for her baby's nursery went unused. For example, she bought a cot bumper, only to learn that they aren't recommended for safety reasons – as babies can overheat or get tangled in the fasteners once they become more mobile. She also bought a changing unit, but found that she preferred to change her baby on a changing mat on the floor. So do bear in mind that a lot of items you'll see in the shops are unnecessary, or even a safety hazard, and if money is short it is best to focus on the key items you and your baby will really need and use. Provided you have the basics to start with, you can always buy extra items as and when you need them.

Clothing

Six to eight all in one suits (babygrows) – perfect for the first three months when your baby will probably hate being dressed and undressed; they are cool enough for the summer and, with the addition of a vest and maybe a cardigan, they are cosy enough for the winter. They have convenient popper fastenings to help you change their nappy quickly and easily.

Fast-growing babies

Remember babies grow quickly, so if anyone offers to buy clothes for your baby suggest they buy bigger sizes, so that you don't end up with more clothes in newborn size than your baby will realistically wear – though of course they will need to bear in mind the changing seasons.

Six to eight vests (bodysuits) – these have envelope necks to make putting them on easy and poppers for easy nappy changes. In the winter they can be worn under an all-in-one and in really hot weather they can be worn alone. You can buy short or long-sleeved versions to suit different times of the year.

Four cardigans or light fleece tops – these provide extra warmth during the winter and on cooler summer days.

One coat or padded all-in-one suit – this is an essential item for winter-born babies but if your baby will spend a lot of time travelling in a car, as well as a pram, make sure you choose one that is not too thick, as your baby may overheat.

Warm mittens – if your baby is due in the winter.

Two hats – woollen or fleece hats for the winter will keep your baby warm when outdoors; remember your baby will lose a lot of heat from their head. For the summer cotton wide-brimmed (fisherman style) or foreign-legion styles will protect your baby's face, ears and neck from the sun[1]. Those with an elasticated or Velcro strap that fits under the chin are great for making sure they stay in place. A couple of cotton jersey pull-on hats are ideal for premature babies, or for cool summer days.

Aim for ease and comfort

Don't feel you have to dress your baby up every day. Choose clothing that's easy to put on and keeps your baby comfortable and not too warm or too cold.

Optional extras

You could get away with dressing your baby in the items listed above, but you may want to add some optional extras such as:

One or two dresses/sets of tops and trousers – these are good for days when you may want to dress up your baby a little.

Four pairs of tights/socks – socks have a tendency to fall off and get lost and if you buy all-in-ones suits, you shouldn't need them. However, if you want your baby to wear a dress or trousers occasionally, you will need some. Tights are ideal for baby girls to wear with dresses on a cold day – though they can be a little tricky to put on!

Two pairs of scratch mittens – these can come in handy if your baby has a tendency to scratch themselves with their nails. However, you might want to wait and see if you need them first.

Washing your baby's clothes

It is a good idea to wash your baby's clothes, even if they are new, in non-biological washing detergent before they wear them – or at least those items that will go next to their delicate skin; this is to remove any dirt or chemicals remaining after their manufacture or transit. Avoid using biological washing liquids/powders or fabric conditioners, as they contain enzymes that could irritate your baby's skin. Opt for a non-biological detergent instead. If your baby's skin seems to be prone to irritation, you could try a detergent designed for sensitive skin, choose one that is free from fragrance and other additives.

Nappy changing

Nappies (a 45-pack of disposable nappies or 20 reusable) – your newborn will need frequent nappy changes – as many as 12 a day – so make sure you buy enough to get you through the first couple of days. However, avoid buying dozens of nappies until you know your baby's weight – a pack of newborn size should suffice initially. There is a huge choice of nappies available, but the main two types are disposable or reusable.

Disposable nappies are the most convenient because you don't have to spend time washing them. They also tend to be more absorbent than cotton nappies, so they don't need changing as often.

On the other hand, according to the National Childbirth Trust (NCT), cotton reusable nappies work out cheaper than disposables – by as much as £900 – depending on which brands you compare (during the period your baby is in nappies) and are more environmentally friendly – if they are washed at 40°C and line dried. If you go for modern fitted cotton nappies rather than terry-towelling ones, they are as easy to put on your baby as disposables. Traditional white square terry-towelling nappies are the cheapest, but you have to fold them to fit your baby and they need to be worn with a nappy liner and plastic pants.

Tip

Reusable nappies don't suit every baby/parent, so buy or borrow one or two at first to try out, otherwise you could waste money.

Basically the decision is down to cost and environmental considerations versus convenience. The choice is yours. However, even if you opt for reusable nappies it is a good idea to keep a pack of disposables in reserve for days when you haven't got any clean or dry reusable ones.

Nappy pail – this is a bucket with a secure-fitting lid where you can store soiled nappies, or soak them in hot soapy water, prior to washing. A nappy pail can also be used as a bin for bagged-up, used disposable nappies – so you don't need to keep dashing out to the wheelie bin so often.

Plastic nappy sacks – soiled nappies smell, so it's a good idea to put them in a bag before you bin them.

Baby wipes – if you intend using them (see page 24). For more information on caring for your baby's skin see page 83.

Barrier or nappy rash cream – a thin layer of cream should be applied to your baby's bottom at every nappy change to prevent and treat nappy rash.

A changing mat – these are usually foam filled with a wipe-clean surface. Some mats come with a removable towel liner but these are usually more expensive and not really necessary. You can also buy lightweight travel changing mats that fold up and have handles, so that you always have a hygienic surface you can change your baby's nappy on when you're out and about.

Breastfeeding equipment

It could be argued that if you plan to breastfeed your baby you won't need any special equipment – however you may find these items useful:

Breast pads – these disposable or reusable cotton pads fit inside your bra cups and absorb any leaking milk.

A breast pump – if you/your partner plan to give your baby breast milk from a bottle at times then an electric or hand breast pump can make expressing milk much faster.

Tip Note: If you are able to express by hand, you won't need a pump.

Two nursing bras – many women manage to breastfeed while wearing a well-fitting, comfortable bra – you can just lift the bra cup up during feeding. However, there are specially designed nursing bras with drop cups for easier access during feeding. They are also designed to give you extra support to the breasts at a time when they are likely to be a cup size or two bigger than usual. You can still wear an underwired bra providing it fits well and doesn't dig in – but they are not quite as easy, or comfortable, to lift up during a feed.

Hypoallergenic lanolin cream for sore or cracked nipples – such as Lansinoh HPA Lanolin, which doesn't need to be wiped off before you feed your baby and has myriad other uses including alleviating nappy rash and dry skin patches and as a balm for dry, cracked lips. Note: lanolin can trigger allergic contact dermatitis in some people, but this brand is recommended by Allergy UK for its significantly reduced allergen content. See the Directory, page 198, for further details.

Bottle-feeding equipment

Six bottles – you can buy inexpensive basic bottles that come in various sizes and can be used in standard bottle warmers, sterilisers and bottle carriers. You can buy anti-colic bottles, which may have a vent or a slow-flow/vented teat to reduce the amount of air your baby swallows when feeding. Some bottles are designed to be sterilised directly in the microwave. You can also buy disposable bottles that are useful for occasional bottle feeds or on a day out. Most major brands of baby bottle are now bisphenol A (BPA) free. BPA is a chemical used in polycarbonate plastics that is thought to disrupt hormones and potentially have a detrimental effect on a baby's growth and development. Another option, if you are concerned about other chemicals used to make plastic baby bottles, is glass feeding bottles, which are made from heat-resistant, toughened glass. The downside of these bottles is that they can shatter if dropped and tend to be much more expensive than plastic ones.

Six teats – a new baby will probably do best on a slow-flow or variflow teat, which allows your baby to control the milk flow in a similar way as they would at the breast. You can buy these both with the bottles and separately.

A bottle and teat brush – all bottles and teats need to be scrubbed and washed before sterilising.

Sterilising equipment – you can choose from electric steam sterilisers, microwave steam sterilisers, and cold-water sterilising units, which are used with sterilising solution (hypochlorite). If you prefer, you can sterilise your baby's feeding equipment by boiling it in a pan, though this will obviously be time-consuming. For more information on sterilising feeding equipment see page 74.

An electric bottle warmer – this is a useful item, though you could just use a jug of hot water instead. You can also buy a bottle-sized travel flask that you fill with hot water before you go out, to warm your baby's bottle when out and about.

Six cotton bibs/muslin cloths – these are useful for catching milk drips, regurgitated milk or dribble during feeds.

Bathing

A baby bath – this can make bath time easier, though it has to be filled and emptied manually and they do take up room, which could be an issue if space is limited. You can also buy baby baths with an extra wide rim that fixes on top of an adult bath. These have a plughole to let the water drain out into the family bath. Choose a sturdy one and make sure you measure your family bath before you buy, to ensure it will fit properly. Another option is a bucket bath, which, as the name suggests, is bucket-shaped to support newborn babies to sit upright, or in a foetal position, so your hands are free to wash your baby.

Alternatively you could buy a newborn bath support, which will enable you to bath them safely in your family bath; this means you can fill and empty the bath as usual and avoid having to carry water around.

Tip Another quick and easy option is to use the washbasin to bath your baby in. To make it safer for your baby, cover the taps with a pair of socks.

Two baby towels – these are useful, but not essential because you could allocate a small bath towel to be used only for your baby instead.

A sponge or flannel – useful for washing your baby, but you may prefer to just use your hands.

Baby toiletries – it is not necessary to buy a lot of toiletries for your baby – especially in the first four weeks, when their skin can be especially sensitive and washing with plain water may be preferable. However, if you would like to use toiletries make sure you choose those especially designed for babies' sensitive skin; there are several brands to choose from, including supermarkets' own branded products; these are all designed to be gentle on your baby's skin – to avoid drying it out or causing irritation.

Baby wipes – having a pack of these can be useful, especially when you are out and about and don't have access to clean warm water. Experts recommend using cotton wool and warm water for the first four weeks – you could moisten some cotton wool balls in water and wrap them up in cling film or pop them in a handy plastic container, but if you prefer the convenience of baby wipes choose fragrance-free, organic or sensitive ones. If your baby develops a rash after using them, you can always revert back to using plain water and cotton wool.

Baby bath/wash – these are usually mild, emollient and pH balanced.

Baby shampoo – choose a mild formula that is designed not to sting the eyes.

You can also buy products that double up as a shampoo and baby wash.

Baby lotion/baby oil – this can be applied to your baby's skin after a bath to prevent their skin from drying out. If your baby develops eczema you may need to see your GP who may recommend using a suitable bath oil and emollient. For more information about treating minor ailments see page 131.

Note: In the first few weeks you may prefer not to use baby cleanser and shampoo on your baby's sensitive skin. However, if your baby's skin can tolerate them, they are effective for washing away traces of poo, stale milk etc. and leave your baby smelling fresh.

Sleeping

When it comes to deciding what type of bed to buy choose the one/s best suited to you and your baby's needs.

Moses basket – in the first few months, while your baby is small, a Moses basket can be good choice; it is smaller than a cot, so your baby will feel more secure in it, and it is lightweight with handles, so it is easy to carry from room to room. You can safely use a Moses basket until your baby is old enough to pull themselves up – usually at around three to four months. Most come with a foam mattress, a padded liner and a cover. You can also buy a stand, which means your baby will be raised up from the floor and the basket can be lined up with your bed for easier access during night feeds.

Safety tip: When buying a Moses basket make sure that the handles are strong and meet in the middle. Always carry the basket with the handles together and support your baby with one hand underneath. If you have any concerns, lift your baby out of the basket before moving it.

When you want your baby to start sleeping in a cot, place them in their Moses basket inside the cot to gradually accustom them to the change.

Carrycot – you can buy these individually, or as part of a travel system, which can save you money – see more about travel systems on page 30. Like Moses baskets they are smaller than a cot, so they are cosier for a newborn to sleep in. If you choose to buy a carrycot that's part of a travel system, check whether you will need to buy a separate mattress if you plan to use it as their main bed, as the mattress needs to be firm enough to support your baby when they are asleep.

Crib – these are usually made of wood and, like a Moses basket, are much smaller than a cot, so they may be more suitable for your newborn. You can also buy models that have a rocking motion – a bonus when trying to get your little one to sleep.

Cot – a cot is much bigger than a Moses basket or crib, so your new baby may look a bit lost when you first put them in it. However, it will last right through until they are ready to go into their own bed, so it is a good option if your budget is tight; you can even buy cots that convert into a toddler bed, which are even better value for money. If you plan to use a cot from the outset then you can also buy a cot divider, which is placed below your baby's feet to stop them from sliding down under the bedding (known as the 'feet to foot' position) – which could otherwise pose a suffocation risk.

Safety guidelines for cots

All new cots for sale in the UK have to conform to safety standard BS EN 716-2:2008. This is to ensure that the cot is deep enough, has bars which are the correct space in between, and has no cut outs or steps. If you buy a second-hand cot make sure it is from a smoke-free home and check that the bars are between 4.5 cm and 6.5 cm apart to ensure baby's head can't slip in between the bars. You should always buy a new mattress and make sure it fits the cot well with no gaps where your baby could become trapped.

Bedding

A lightweight, cotton jersey or cotton wrap (blanket) is useful to make your baby feel secure without overheating during the early weeks.

Four sheets – to fit the pram, crib, Moses basket or cot. Sheets are also useful for swaddling your newborn to help them settle.

Four lightweight pram-size blankets – to fit a pram, crib, or Moses basket.

Cot-size lightweight blanket – if you are putting your baby in a cot from birth.

Baby sleeping bag – these are recommended for safer sleeping and can be useful if your baby tends to kick off their covers. You can buy them with or without sleeves.

Safety guidelines for bedding

Avoid using a quilt, as your baby could overheat. Use a sheet, a lightweight blanket or a sleeping bag instead. Place your baby in the 'feet-to-foot' position (feet touching the foot of the cot) and tuck the sheets/blanket in firmly – no higher than your baby's shoulders, so they can't slip underneath and suffocate. Don't use a pillow or cot bumper and remove any soft toys before putting your baby down to sleep.

It's best to buy a sleeping bag after your baby is born, so you can make sure it fits properly around their neck and they can't slip down inside. Never use a sleeping bag with a blanket over the top, as your baby could overheat. Choose a low-tog bag for summer (0.5 tog or 1 tog) and no more than a 2.5 tog for winter – a higher tog could make your baby too hot. Always take the temperature of the room into account, not just the season and remember that being too cold is just as dangerous for your baby as being too hot.

Transport

A baby carrier (sling) – this can be invaluable, especially in the first three months. It is an easy way to carry your baby when you need to pop out to the shops, or if you just want to go for a walk. It's also ideal for carrying your baby around the house while you do a few light chores. If your baby is fretful and won't go to sleep, you will probably find they will settle in the carrier, as the movement and sound of your heartbeat will remind them of when they were in the womb and have a soothing effect, which will help them to drop off. You will need to decide whether to buy a carrier that will last until your baby is a toddler, or one designed for a newborn. Bear in mind that you might struggle to carry your baby as they get heavier. Choose a model with wide, well-padded shoulder straps for comfort. If both you and your partner will be using the baby carrier, pick one that can be adjusted to fit you both. If you plan to use the carrier outdoors opt for one with a canopy to protect their head from the sun and rain.

A pram, pushchair or buggy that lies flat – as a newborn baby needs to lie flat for at least the first three months, or ideally until they are able to sit up themselves – usually at four to seven months. This is to ensure their backs and necks are fully supported and can develop normally. Before buying a pram, pushchair or buggy check the frame is sturdy and the brakes work properly. You should also make sure the handles are the right height for you.

A car seat – also called a safety restraint. You must always put your baby in their seat when travelling in a car. It is both illegal and dangerous to carry your baby in your arms in a vehicle. The safest way for a baby weighing up to 28 lb 11 oz (13 kg) to travel is in a rear-facing infant car seat on the front or back seat. Rear-facing car seats protect the baby's head, neck and spine better than forward-facing seats, so it's best to keep your baby in a rear-facing car seat until they are heavier than the maximum weight for the baby seat (usually by about 15 months), or the top of their head is above the top of the seat. After that it is safe to use a forward-facing model. Make sure your car seat is fitted properly. Never put a rear-facing infant car seat in a front or rear seat fitted with an air bag, unless it has been deactivated. Never buy a second-hand car seat – it may have been damaged in an accident. When buying a car seat look for the United Nations ECE Regulation number R44/04.

A travel system – this consists of a car seat, carrycot and pram, pushchair or buggy and is a cost-effective option. The car seat and carrycot both click into the pushchair, which means you don't have to disturb your baby when transporting them while they are asleep. You can also use the carrycot for your baby to sleep in for the first few months instead of a Moses basket. As with car seats it is advisable not to buy a second-hand travel system in case the car seat has been damaged. Also be aware that they can be quite bulky, which might be an issue if you have a small hallway or car, or limited storage space.

A rain cover – you should buy one that is designed to fit the particular model of pram, pushchair, or buggy where possible.

A sunshade/or pram parasol – if it is summer – to protect your baby from the sun. Experts advise keeping your baby out of direct sunlight until the age of six months.

A changing bag – you'll need a good-sized bag to hold all the items you need to take with you whenever you leave the house. Some bags open out into a changing mat, while others come with a separate changing mat that fits inside the bag. Most have separate pockets and compartments to store wet wipes, nappies, spare baby clothes and feeding bottles. However, if you already have a large handbag or beach bag, that would do. For a checklist of what to take with you when you go out see page 100.

A thermal bottle holder – this will keep your baby's bottle/s of formula or expressed milk cold when you go out and about.

Useful extras

Six muslin squares – you can use these instead of a bib to protect your baby's clothing during feeds, or your own clothing when burping your baby; you can put them on the changing mat to make the surface more comfortable when nappy changing; you can use them moistened with water to clean your baby when out and about; you can tie a knot in one end to make a comforter.

A baby monitor – this enables you to listen to, or see, your baby when they are in a different room. You can also buy sensory monitors that pick up your baby's movements and breathing; when none are detected for a very short period an alarm goes off.

A baby bouncer – this is a soft, bouncy seat that can be used from birth. The basic models are fairly inexpensive and are ideal to put your baby in when they are awake, but you need your hands free; they are light and easy to carry, so you can take your baby with you to any room in the house. Your baby can see what is going on around them, so it keeps them amused. I found them ideal when I was hungry, but my baby was awake – I could keep them close to me and rock them gently using one foot, while my hands were free for me to be able to eat. Quite often the gentle rocking motion would send them to sleep.

Sun blinds for the car – if you can afford them these are a useful but optional extra to protect your baby's eyes from sun glare.

A basic baby's first aid kit

As your baby won't be mobile yet they are unlikely to suffer bumps or cuts, so a basic first aid kit at this age should be designed to deal with the minor ailments your baby is likely to suffer from such as wind and colic, nappy rash and other minor skin irritations and fevers.

Below are some suggestions as to what you could include in your baby's first aid kit for the first three months:

- ▶ **Saline nasal spray** – to ease a blocked nose (vapour rubs can only be used from three months)

- ▶ **A digital baby thermometer** – for a fast, accurate temperature reading

- ▶ **Liquid pain relief** – (from two months onwards) such as infant paracetamol

- ▶ **An oral syringe** – to measure and administer liquid pain relief or medicine

▸ **Calamine lotion** – to soothe minor skin irritations, rashes and insect bites

▸ **Almond oil** – to treat dry skin patches/cradle cap (scaly patches on scalp) or for baby massage

 Note: Gripe water is commonly used to relieve colic but it must not be given to babies under one month old.

For some tips on treating minor ailments and emergency first aid for babies see pages 131.

CHAPTER 2

FEED YOUR BABY

Breastfeeding is the way nature intended mothers to nourish their babies and offers many benefits to both mum and child, but it isn't always plain sailing and doesn't suit everyone. What is most important is that your baby is well-fed and content and you are happy with the feeding method you have chosen. Although breast milk is the perfect food for your baby, there are some excellent formula feeds that closely replicate mothers' milk, so no one should feel guilty if they decide against breastfeeding, or find they cannot breast feed for whatever reason.

This chapter aims to help mums make an informed decision about whether to breastfeed or bottle-feed by explaining the benefits of breastfeeding and how it works; this information will also help you to understand the advice on how to breastfeed and how to prevent and overcome common problems. It also suggests ways partners can still be involved in breastfeeding – both by providing practical support and by feeding their baby expressed milk from a bottle. In addition there's information on formula milks and how to bottle-feed, as well as how to combine breast and bottle-feeding.

In this chapter:

► Resolve the breastfeeding versus bottle-feeding dilemma
► Breastfeeding pros and cons
► What's in breast milk?

- ▶ Diet and breastfeeding
- ▶ How breastfeeding works
- ▶ Starting breastfeeding
- ▶ Keeping going – common breastfeeding concerns
- ▶ How to express your milk
- ▶ How to combine breast and bottle-feeding
- ▶ How to overcome common breastfeeding problems
- ▶ Real-life experiences of two breastfeeding mums
- ▶ Bottle-feeding pros and cons
- ▶ Types of infant formula
- ▶ How to sterilise feeding equipment
- ▶ How to mix a bottle of formula
- ▶ How to give your baby a bottle
- ▶ Bottle-feeding dos and don'ts
- ▶ How to burp your baby

Resolve the breastfeeding versus bottle-feeding dilemma

Some mothers are determined to breastfeed, no matter what, some are ambivalent and some really don't want to do it. Making the choice between breast- or bottle-feeding can be quite emotional – you want to do what is best for your baby and breastfeeding is widely encouraged and accepted as the best option for your baby; but perhaps you have misgivings about it, or you may try it and then find that it just doesn't suit you, for whatever reason.

If you are determined to breastfeed and manage to overcome any early difficulties and keep going you will be glad you did, as you should find that it gets easier as the weeks go by and knowing that you are feeding your baby yourself can give you a real sense of achievement.

If you can't decide either way, it never hurts to attempt breastfeeding. You may find that you and your baby take to it easily and, even if it doesn't work out in the long-term, they will at least have benefitted from your nutrient and antibody-rich colostrum ('early milk').

If you decide to breastfeed, but then find it's making you miserable, or your baby isn't thriving, then bottle-feeding is probably the better option for you both. However, bear in mind that a lot of initial breastfeeding problems can be resolved and once you stop nursing your milk will quickly dry up, so persevere if you can and only give up if you are sure that is the right choice for you. Another option is mixed feeding – i.e. combining breast- and bottle-feeding – that way your baby will still benefit from your breast milk, but feeding them formula as well can take some of the pressure off you. It can also make things easier, if at any stage you need to leave your baby in the care of others.

However, if you start breastfeeding and then find you are unable to continue, or decide that it really isn't for you – please don't feel guilty, or think that you have failed as a mother. What really matters is that your baby is loved and well cared for – they will still thrive on formula.

To help you make an informed choice between breastfeeding and bottle-feeding and understand this chapter's advice, we'll discuss the pros and cons of breastfeeding versus bottle-feeding; we'll then look at what breast milk contains, how breastfeeding works and how to overcome common worries and problems, before focussing on formula milks and how to bottle-feed.

Breastfeeding pros and cons

The decision whether or not to breastfeed is a personal one for mums; to help you decide whether to give it a go here are some breastfeeding pros and cons.

Pros

It is free – though you will need some equipment – such as breast pads to absorb leaks, a breast pump if you intend to express milk – though this can be done manually – and one or two bottles to feed your baby the expressed milk.

It is the perfect food and drink for your baby – with exactly the right amount of protein, fat, carbohydrates and nutrients as well as immunity-boosting prebiotics and antibodies that protect against illnesses and allergies. Your baby shouldn't need additional formula or fluids provided you feed them on demand and they are feeding well.

It doesn't need any preparation – sterilising of bottles, mixing of formula, warming up, storage and so on – so it is always available on demand.

If you breastfeed, your baby is less likely to suffer from illness – such as tummy bugs, ear and respiratory infections and allergies – because of the prebiotics and antibodies it contains. Recent research shows that it can even protect your baby from obesity, heart disease and diabetes in later life.

Breastfeeding helps you regain your figure quicker – because it releases the 'cuddle hormone' oxytocin, which makes the uterus contract and go back to its original size and position sooner than in non-breastfeeding mothers. It can also help you lose the body fat stored up during pregnancy, as you need 500 or more extra calories per day to produce milk.

Breastfeeding reduces your risk of breast and ovarian cancer – because it cuts your exposure to the female hormones oestrogen and progesterone, which are involved in the development of these cancers.

Breastfeeding ensures you sit down and relax regularly every day – and gives you the confidence of knowing you are giving your baby the best start in life.

Cons

Only you can breastfeed your baby – unless of course you express your milk – so you are 'on call' 24 hours a day.

You might feel embarrassed about breastfeeding your baby in public – though there are now several schemes that encourage private, public and voluntary organisations to offer more 'breastfeeding-friendly' facilities. See also 'Keeping going – common breastfeeding concerns' on page 46.

Breast milk can be low in vitamin D – due to UK mothers' lack of exposure to sunlight. The NHS advises breastfeeding mothers to take 10 mg of vitamin D daily to prevent babies being deficient.

Even though it's *natural* it won't necessarily come *naturally* – to you or your baby. It takes time for you and your baby to learn how to do it properly.

What's in breast milk?

Human breast milk contains exactly the right balance of nutrients for a baby's optimum health, growth and development, including:

Water – is the main component of breast milk. So a breastfed baby gets enough fluids from their feeds and doesn't need extra water – even in hot weather.

Easy-to-digest proteins – which means your baby absorbs nearly all of the protein in breast milk, which is why their stools are much less bulky than those of bottle-fed babies, and explains why breastfed babies need feeding more often.

Fats – including omega-3 and 6 essential fatty acids (EFAs) that are important for the development of your baby's eyes and brain.

Carbohydrates – in the form of lactose (milk sugar) which helps the baby absorb calcium and other sugars called oligosaccharides; these act as a prebiotics which prevent infections by promoting the growth of *lactobacilli* ('good' bacteria) and preventing 'bad' bacteria from sticking to the throat and gut linings.

Vitamins – including vitamins A, C and D; however if a breastfeeding mother doesn't get outdoors in sunlight regularly they may need a vitamin D supplement.

Minerals – such as calcium, which is absorbed more easily due to the lactose in the milk, and iron in the form of lactoferrin, which also helps prevent infections.

Probiotics ('good' bacteria) – including various types of *lactobacilli*, which help to prevent illnesses like gastroenteritis.

Antibodies – breast milk contains immunoglobulin A (IgA), a protein designed to protect the baby from all the bacterial, viral and fungal infections the mother may have suffered from such as gastroenteritis, colds and flu. Breast milk also contains other live cells that protect babies from infections.

Diet and breastfeeding

You don't need to eat a special diet to breastfeed successfully. Research shows that what a breastfeeding mother eats has little effect on the composition of her breast milk. However, if your diet doesn't supply enough nutrients for milk production your body will raid those stored in your body, which could leave you lacking in certain vitamins and minerals and affect *your* well-being, rather than your baby's. To stay healthy, try to eat a balanced diet that includes whole grains, fish, lean meat, dairy foods, nuts, seeds and fruit and vegetables. Drink plenty of fluids, but watch your caffeine and alcohol intake as these pass into your milk and could affect your baby.

The only time you may need to adjust your diet is if your baby displays signs of cow's milk allergy (CMA) triggered by cow's milk proteins being passed on through your milk – for more information on CMA see page 73. If you suspect your baby has CMA from your breast milk you could try cutting out dairy products from your diet for a couple of weeks to see if their symptoms improve. However, to avoid a calcium deficiency you would need to eat alternative sources such as sardines eaten with the bones, almonds, Brazil nuts, dried apricots, dates, figs, seeds, green leafy vegetables, tofu or soya milk products. If you eat well, the only supplement you are likely to need is vitamin D, as in the UK it is difficult to get enough of the main source – sunlight on the skin. You can find out more about eating well in Chapter 8, on page 183.

How breastfeeding works

Breastfeeding involves a series of mechanisms that result in milk being produced and released into the milk ducts so that your baby can drink it. Here is the lowdown on how breastfeeding works.

Prolactin – the hormone that stimulates milk production – increases after the birth and is produced every time your baby feeds from your breasts. Your baby's sucking action also makes your breasts more sensitive and responsive to prolactin. So the more often you feed your baby the more prolactin – and therefore the more milk – you will produce.

Colostrum – is the thick, yellowish milk your breasts produce towards the end of pregnancy and for the first few days after the birth. It is rich in vitamins and minerals, as well as antibodies and white blood cells to protect against infections. It also has more protein and less sugar and fat than the 'proper' milk that comes later.

Transitional milk – is produced as your breasts gradually replace colostrum with more mature milk. Transitional milk looks milkier and provides your baby with more fat and sugar than colostrum.

Mature milk – has about a fifth of the amount of protein of colostrum and consists of foremilk and hindmilk.

Foremilk – is released at the beginning of each feed. It is quite watery and thirst quenching and is always available 'on tap' whenever your baby wants to feed.

Hindmilk – is much richer than foremilk, as it contains more fat. It remains in the milk glands until it is 'let down' into the milk ducts either at the start of the feed, or within a minute or so of your baby starting to suck.

Letdown reflex – this is where the hindmilk, which is stored in the milk glands, floods into the milk ducts, so that your baby can feed from it. The 'cuddle-hormone' oxytocin stimulates letdown; your body releases oxytocin in response to cues such as your baby crying, or even when you think about your baby – especially if you haven't fed them for some time and your breasts are full of milk. Oxytocin can also be released when your baby starts feeding from the breast. You will feel the milk rushing in and a tingling or warmth in your breasts during letdown, or you might experience milk leaking or dripping from your breasts. A reliable letdown reflex can take a week or two to establish. It's a fairly sensitive mechanism that can be affected by stress and anxiety – which is why breastfeeding mums are advised to take things as easy as possible during the first few weeks of breastfeeding. The more often you feed your baby the quicker you'll establish a dependable letdown reflex.

Your baby gets your milk using three actions – by sucking to pull your nipple and areola into their mouth, by milking – which involves squeezing the nipple and areola (the darker area around your nipple) with their tongue to release the milk and by swallowing the milk as it sprays into the back of their mouth. Your milk lets down in spurts – in between these your baby will continue to suck in short, sharp bursts to stimulate the milk flow.

Starting breastfeeding

Below are some key steps to starting breastfeeding.

Feed your baby as soon after the birth as you can – your baby's sucking action will stimulate your breasts to produce milk and encourage your womb to start contracting back to its normal size and position. You can usually start breastfeeding straight after your baby is born. Your baby's suckling instinct will be strongest in the first hour, so putting your baby to your breast as soon as you can will get your breastfeeding off to a good start.

Make yourself comfortable – so that you feel relaxed, which, as explained, is essential for successful breastfeeding. You may find resting your supporting arm on the armrest of a settee or chair or on one or two cushions helps. To help you unwind you may want to watch TV, listen to music, or read a book. You may find you feel thirsty when you are feeding your baby, so it's useful to have a glass of water to hand.

Position your baby correctly – the cradle hold is the one most mums adopt naturally and involves cradling your baby in the arm that is on the same side as the breast you're feeding from, with their head resting in the crook of your elbow. Hold them close to you with their whole body facing you and their chin against your breast. Your baby's nose should be opposite your nipple and their ear, shoulder and hip should all be aligned. The cross-cradle hold is also popular with new mums because it enables you to guide your baby onto your breast more easily. Here you cradle your baby across the front of your body, using the arm *opposite* the nursing breast. Always hold your baby so you are supporting their back and shoulders, but ensure you are not touching the back of their head, because they will need to be able to tip their head back. If you support your baby's back and shoulders their head will still be well controlled. You might find it helpful to use a cushion or pillow to help raise your baby to the right level; you can buy L-shaped breastfeeding cushions that can help you to position your baby correctly. In the first day or two after the birth a midwife will be on-hand to help you find the best position to get breastfeeding off to a good start.

Tip: Remember the breastfeeding mantra: 'nose to nipple, tummy to mummy'.

Make sure your baby latches on properly – as soon as they open their mouth wide bring it towards your breast, with their chin touching your breast first. Once your baby is attached more of your areola (the darker skin around your nipple) should be showing above your baby's top lip than below their bottom lip. Their chin should be pushed into your breast and their cheeks should look full and rounded. You should feel your baby sucking and swallowing.

When your baby finishes feeding from the first breast offer the other – babies can take anywhere from 10 to 20 minutes to empty the first breast – though some take more or less time than that – every baby is different. If they don't want to feed from the second breast that's OK – just offer it first next time to ensure each breast is emptied. However, in the early days it's a good idea to swap breasts every 10 minutes or so, to ensure both breasts are equally stimulated to produce milk. If you offer your second breast and your baby either doesn't want to feed from it, or only feeds for a short time, offer that one first next time, to ensure both breasts are emptied regularly. Some babies like to comfort suck on the breast after they've emptied it – rather like a bottle-fed baby might suck on a dummy or their thumb. There's no reason to stop this unless you have sore nipples, or need to do something else.

Feed on demand – to stimulate your breasts to produce enough milk for your baby's needs and ensure they are well-nourished and hydrated.

Recognise when your baby wants to feed – they will let you know when they are hungry with a series of cues; initially they might start mouthing i.e. opening and closing their mouth, or sucking their hand or fist. They may then start rooting for the breast – turning their head and opening and closing their mouth and trying to suck on anything within reach! If these hunger signals go unheeded your baby will usually start crying.

Go with the flow – in the early days especially, when your baby may want to feed most of the time, with few gaps in between. Don't panic and think they aren't getting enough milk – their stomach is quite small, so they will naturally need to feed little and often; remember every time your baby feeds they will stimulate milk production. To help you relax and enjoy feeding and getting to know your baby ask your partner or another family member to take over essential chores.

Avoid giving a bottle or dummy in the early days – as the technique your baby uses to feed from a bottle or suck on a dummy is completely different to the one they use to breastfeed, so this could confuse them and make it harder for them to feed from your breast. If you need to, you could introduce them at about six weeks, when your baby should have settled into a breastfeeding routine.

Keeping going – common breastfeeding concerns

Breastfeeding doesn't always run smoothly and in the early days you may worry that you're not doing it right, or your baby isn't getting enough milk. The key to long-term success is to persevere and overcome your concerns and deal with any problems. Worrying that you aren't feeding your baby correctly, or you're not producing enough milk to satisfy their needs, can affect your milk production and flow. As you will see below many concerns about breastfeeding are unfounded, so try not to get stressed and learn to enjoy the process.

I'm not sure if I'm feeding my baby correctly

If your baby appears satisfied and is gaining weight, you are feeding your baby correctly. In the early weeks your midwife and health visitor will monitor your baby's weight and will let you know if there is a problem. However, if you still have concerns about breastfeeding you can discuss them with your midwife, health visitor or a breastfeeding counsellor.

I'm worried I'm not producing enough milk

Most concerns about not producing enough milk are unfounded and tend to be based on things that aren't really related such as:

My baby wants to feed all the time – rather than showing that you don't have enough milk this could be down to a number of things including the fact that your baby's stomach is small, which means they need small, frequent feeds – especially in the early days; it could also mean your baby is having a growth spurt, or your baby is cluster feeding – see 'How to overcome common breastfeeding problems', page 56. Remember every baby is different and just because someone else's baby is going x number of hours between feeds doesn't mean that yours will as well.

My breasts aren't leaking milk – not every mother leaks milk and even those that do find that their breasts leak less and less as time goes on.

My breasts feel soft – in the early days your breasts are likely to feel full and hard, but as time goes on they become more efficient at producing just the right amount of milk for your baby; also an emptier breast means more milk will be produced.

Your baby only feeds for a few minutes – rather than being a sign that you aren't making enough milk, this could simply be due to your baby being very efficient at getting the milk quickly and your milk flowing quite fast. Again all babies are individuals – some are fast feeders and some take much longer to get the amount of milk they need.

I have small breasts – the size of your breasts has no bearing on their ability to produce milk, or how much milk you will produce.

My baby won't settle after a feed – if your baby won't settle when you put them down to sleep after a feed it could be because they were nice and warm and comfortable snuggled into your breast and the Moses basket or cot doesn't feel quite as cosy, rather than because they didn't get enough milk. Or they may just want to be held or be able to suck from the breast for comfort, rather than to satisfy hunger.

I can't express much milk – some women manage to express milk quite easily, others find it quite difficult to squeeze out even a couple of ounces. Rather than 'proving' you don't have much milk, it could be down to the fact that you can only let down milk when your baby is feeding from you.

Signs of insufficient milk

While not having enough milk is not usually the problem, it's important that you are aware of the signs that you really aren't producing enough milk, so that you can make a decision about how to proceed. The signs of insufficient milk are as follows.

Your baby fails to gain weight – your baby will lose weight just after they are born and should regain their birth weight by about two weeks. After that they should gain about 150 to 200 g a week in the first three months or so. If your baby loses more than a tenth of their birth weight it could be a cause for concern, but bear in mind they may have been bloated with fluids when they were first born. This can happen for several reasons – for example if you were put on a drip during labour. Initially your midwife and then your health visitor will monitor your baby's weight and let you know if they have any concerns.

Trust your own instincts too – you will know if your baby isn't putting on weight. If there are concerns, your health visitor or midwife might want to check that your baby is latching on and feeding properly. Check your breastfeeding technique – are you offering your baby the second breast after they have emptied the first, to make sure they are getting enough milk? You may need to feed your baby more often – the more milk they take the more you should produce. Try not to get stressed about breastfeeding as this is more likely to cause problems.

The support you can expect after the birth

Your community midwife will visit you at home, usually on the day you are discharged from hospital. She will weigh your baby to check they are feeding well and make sure their umbilical cord stump is healing properly. She'll also feel your tummy to make sure your uterus is starting to shrink back to normal. If you had a Caesarean section or any tears or cuts during the birth she will check the wound is healing well. When your baby is five days old your midwife, or a support worker, will ask your consent to do the Newborn Blood Spot Screening, which involves collecting four drops of blood from your baby's heel to screen for nine different disorders, including cystic fibrosis and hypothyroidism; these should be explained to you in detail first.

When your baby is ten to 21 days old, your health visitor will take over the care of you and your baby. On her first home visit she will check your baby's general growth, health and development. She will assess your emotional health with some questions, or a questionnaire. She will also offer advice on establishing your baby's feeding and sleep routines and deal with any queries or concerns. She will ask you to have your baby weighed weekly at your local health clinic or GP's surgery. If you or your baby has any issues, such as postnatal illness (PNI) or colic, she will make further visits. Otherwise your next check-up will take place at six to eight weeks either with her at your home or clinic, or with your GP. During this visit if your health visitor/GP is happy with your baby's progress they may suggest your baby is weighed fortnightly. They will also re-assess your emotional well-being; if they suspect you are depressed your GP should offer you appropriate treatment to help you recover.

Your baby doesn't wee and poo their nappies regularly – if your baby is taking in plenty of milk they will produce wet nappies six to eight times a day and do regular poos.

When to seek medical advice – if your baby isn't producing six to eight wet nappies every 24 hours, if they aren't pooing regularly, or don't seem to be feeding often enough, or putting on weight, see a health professional as soon as possible, as babies who don't get enough milk can become dehydrated quite quickly.

I'm worried about breastfeeding in public

Feeding your baby when out and about seems to be a common concern among breastfeeding mums that can lead to them either giving up, or becoming isolated because they are frightened to leave the house in case their baby needs a feed. The main issue seems to be that many mums are too embarrassed to feed their babies in front of strangers. This isn't helped by the fact that some people disapprove of women breastfeeding in public places – even though it's the most natural thing in the world. Sadly, many shops, cafes and restaurants fail to offer somewhere private, comfortable and hygienic where mums can breastfeed their babies and sometimes the only option is to breastfeed in the toilets. Below are some strategies to help you breastfeed in public.

Preserve your modesty – while you can't change other people's attitudes, you *can* reduce your embarrassment by breastfeeding your baby as discreetly as possible; if you're not displaying any flesh people will be less likely to notice and if they do, they will have no reason to be offended!

Rachel, first-time mum of Emily, told me: 'I'd recommend wearing a nursing bra with a drop cup, along with a vest and a baggy top; you can pull the bra cup and vest down and lift the baggy top up, so you can be a bit more discreet when breastfeeding. Muslin squares were also great for preserving my modesty.' You can buy vests especially designed to make breastfeeding more private and there are baby slings that can be adjusted to allow you to breastfeed your baby discreetly. For more information see the Directory, page 198.

Feed expressed breast milk from a bottle – if you would rather not breastfeed in public you can take a bottle of expressed breast milk in a cool bag with an ice pack to keep it cold. You could also take a flask of hot water and a jug to warm it, but most cafes and restaurants will provide a jug of hot water on request. See also 'How to express your milk' on page 53.

Look for baby-friendly venues – councils across the UK are now encouraging shops, cafes, restaurants, GP surgeries, children's centres, libraries and leisure centres to be more breastfeeding friendly by encouraging them to earn the Breastfeeding Welcome Award. To achieve the award organisations have to meet certain criteria such as making breastfeeding mums welcome in public areas of their premises and providing a clean, comfortable, private space for breastfeeding and baby-changing facilities. Some local councils provide details of baby-friendly organisations and businesses in their area. There are also organisations such as Babies Welcome to help you find baby-friendly venues near you. For more information see the Directory, page 198. There is also a phone app called Feed-Finder that can help you find a breastfeeding-friendly venue when you are out and about. For more details see Useful Products, page 194.

> ### Breastfeeding in public and the law
>
> The Equality Act 2010 made it illegal for anyone to ask a breastfeeding woman to leave a public place such as a cafe, shop or public transport.

What if someone else is looking after my baby?

Again, you could express some milk and leave it in a bottle for whoever is looking after your baby to give to them.

How to express your milk

You can express your milk by hand, with a hand pump or an electric pump. Expressing by hand can work well, but a hand pump can speed up the process and an electric pump would be better still if you need to do a lot of expressing. Electric pumps can be expensive but some of the cheaper models can be just as effective – check the online reviews before you choose; you can also hire a hospital-grade electric pump from the NCT, but if you were to do this on a long-term basis it could be costly. For more details see the Directory, page 198.

Expressing by hand

1. Wash your hands thoroughly.

2. Get a clean sterilised container to express your milk into.

3. Make yourself comfortable.

4. Find your milk ducts. These are about 2.5 cm away from your nipple where your breast tissue has a different texture.

5. With your thumb and fingers in a C-shape gently squeeze your milk ducts and then release. Continue squeezing and releasing rhythmically. You may just get drips at first but if you keep up the milking action you should be rewarded with squirts of milk.

6. If the flow of milk slows down, reposition your fingers slightly to drain the milk from all the ducts. Then change to your other breast and start the process again. Keep alternating breasts until the milk flow stops completely.

When to express

Most mothers find it's best to express straight after feeding their baby so they can collect any leftover milk. This is also a great way to boost your milk supply. Some women find their milk sprays from one breast while their baby is feeding from the other so they can collect that milk. You will usually have more milk earlier on in the day, so you might find it is best to express milk in the morning. But you could try different times to see what works best for you.

How much you can expect to express

The amount you express will vary and it might only be one or two ounces to start with. Use a different clean, sterile container every time, unless you express more than once a day, in which case you can cool the latest batch and add it to the previous one. You could end up having to use the contents of several containers to produce a full feed for your baby.

Storing your milk

Freshly expressed breast milk will keep for up to 6 hours at room temperature (no more than 25˚C). If you won't be using your expressed milk within that time store it in the fridge or the freezer straight away in any clean, sterilised container such as a bottle with a screw cap, a specially designed breast milk storage pot or pre-sterilised bags. Stick a label with the date and time on each container before storing the milk, so that you know when it needs to be used by.

Because breast milk contains anti-infective agents you can store it safely in a fridge for up to five days, so long as your fridge remains at less than 4°C. If the temperature is higher than 4°C, or you don't know the temperature, it is safer to use the milk within three days.

If you want to keep the milk for longer you will need to store it in the freezer – you can buy breast milk storage bags for this purpose. You can keep it for up to two weeks in a freezer compartment and up to six months in a freezer that maintains a temperature of –18°C or less. If you intend to refrigerate or freeze your milk but don't have access to a fridge or freezer straight away, you can store your milk in a cool bag with ice packs until you get home.

Thaw frozen breast milk in the fridge or at room temperature. If thawed in the fridge it can be kept there safely for up to 12 hours. If you need to use the frozen milk straight away hold the container under a warm running tap, or place it in a jug of warm water. Always use milk defrosted in this way as soon as it has thawed fully – otherwise throw it away. Never defrost milk in a microwave or refreeze it. Once your baby has started drinking from a bottle you should discard any unused breast milk after one hour to avoid the risk of your baby picking up a tummy bug. See also 'How to give your baby a bottle' on page 79.

How to overcome common breastfeeding problems

The first few weeks of breastfeeding are the toughest; if you can manage to deal with problems and soldier on you'll probably find that things gradually become easier and easier until breastfeeding is something you do without having to think about it too much; plus you'll enjoy the convenience of having milk that is always available whenever your baby wants it, and without the hassle of having to prepare feeds. Below are some common problems you may experience with suggestions on how to overcome them.

Engorged breasts

When your mature milk first comes in on around day four your breasts might feel swollen, painful and engorged with too much milk. The engorgement should gradually ease as they adjust to producing the right amount of milk for your baby. In the meantime, the best way to relieve engorgement is to feed your baby frequently, making sure they latch on properly. If your breasts are too full and hard for your baby to latch onto, express a little milk before each feed – you can store it in the fridge or freezer for later. Or you could try using nipple shields, which may make it easier for your baby to feed.

If your breasts feel uncomfortably full in between feeds you can express and store the milk for later. If the engorgement is making it too painful to breastfeed, you could use a pump to empty your breasts and feed the expressed milk to your baby from a bottle until it settles down. Try putting warm flannels on your breasts first, to encourage your milk to start flowing.

> ### Try cabbage leaves!
>
> An old-fashioned but clinically proven remedy for relieving engorgement is to put cold cabbage leaves into your bra. Cabbages are rich in sulphur, which is known to reduce swelling and inflammation. The leaves are also thought to reduce milk supply. Wash and dry the leaves first and crush slightly between your fingers to help release the sulphur. Make sure each breast is completely covered. Change the leaves every 2 or 3 hours. If you need to wear breast pads to soak up any leaking milk place them between the cabbage leaves and your bra. Stop using the cabbage leaves as soon as the engorgement settles down, as prolonged use could result in you producing insufficient milk for your baby. If you prefer a less messy remedy you can buy special gel pads from your pharmacist.

Sore nipples

Sore nipples are fairly common when you first start breastfeeding, however, the soreness should go after the first few days as your nipples 'toughen up'. If the problem continues there could be a number of causes:

Your baby isn't latching on properly

This is the most common cause of sore nipples[2]. If your baby doesn't latch on properly, the nipple will be at the front of their mouth rather than the back, so when they suck the nipple will be pulled in and out of their mouth, leading to soreness. Also, your baby won't be able to milk the ducts properly, which will affect your milk flow and production. So if you have sore nipples beyond the first few days, always check that your baby is taking a large mouthful of breast, so that your nipple is at the back of their mouth and they are milking the ducts behind the nipple as they feed. Once your baby starts latching on correctly your nipples should heal and the pain should gradually disappear. To help speed up the healing you could try expressing a little milk at the end of each feed, applying it to your sore nipples and allowing it to dry. This traditional remedy is thought to work because breast milk contains substances that encourage cell growth and prevent infection.

Alternatively you could use nipple shields to protect your nipples during feeds, or express a few feeds, to give your nipples a chance to heal. Another option is to use a nipple cream such as Lansinoh For more information see page 21.

Tongue tie

Tongue tie – where the baby's tongue is attached to the bottom of the mouth by a small piece of skin – is one of the possible reasons your baby isn't latching on properly. Signs of tongue tie include your baby not being able to latch on well and frequent feeding with little weight gain. If you suspect your baby has tongue tie ask your midwife, health visitor or doctor to check. The condition can be corrected with minor surgery, known as a frenulotomy, which involves cutting the tight piece of skin using sterile, sharp, round-ended scissors without the need for an anaesthetic. It is thought that most babies feel little pain and some even sleep through the procedure.

Thrush

If you develop sore nipples along with severe burning, shooting or stabbing pains in your breasts, you may have a thrush infection[3]. Thrush is caused by overgrowth of the fungus/yeast known as *Candida albicans* that normally exists in your body without causing any problem. If you have thrush on your nipples it is likely your baby will have it in their mouth too. Thrush thrives in warm, moist conditions, so your nipples and your baby's mouth provide the perfect breeding ground. As you and your baby will be able to pass the infection to and from each other, you will both need to be treated. If you suspect you or your baby have thrush see your doctor immediately. They will be able to prescribe an antifungal treatment for you and your baby.

Cracked nipple

Sometimes a sore nipple can develop a crack. The best prevention is to treat a sore nipple before it gets any worse, as a cracked nipple can lead to a breast infection known as mastitis (see below). Applying a hypoallergenic lanolin cream such as Lansinoh HPA to your nipple will moisturise it and help it heal. If the pain is severe you may want to take a painkiller such as paracetamol or ibuprofen about half an hour before a feed (not aspirin, as this could cause Reye's Syndrome in your baby – see the table on page 173 for more information about painkillers). You might want to gently express your milk and feed it to your baby from a bottle until the crack has healed.

Mastitis

Mastitis is where the breast tissues become inflamed or infected. The inflamed areas will look red and feel sore, hot and swollen. You may also develop flu-like symptoms such as fever, fatigue, aching and a headache, if an infection develops. You might also feel a lump, known as a blocked duct, caused by a build-up of milk. In fact a build-up of milk is the most common cause of mastitis and is usually due to your breast producing more milk than your baby is taking. It can happen if you miss a feed, or there is a long gap between feeds. It can also be due to your baby not latching on properly which means they don't empty your breasts, or because you have avoided feeding on one side because of a sore nipple, which leads to engorgement and a blocked duct

Giving your baby a dummy or a bottle could also cause mastitis by reducing the amount of time your baby spends at the breast. A cracked nipple can sometimes cause mastitis by allowing an infection into the breast. Other causes include wearing over tight clothing or an injury to your breast.

First-time mums are more likely to develop mastitis, though experienced breastfeeding mums can also get it. It's most likely to happen in the first few weeks of breastfeeding when your breasts are adjusting to your baby's needs.

How to ease mastitis

Although you will find it painful, it's best to keep on feeding your baby as often as possible from the affected breast, making sure they are positioned well and latched on properly. See 'Starting breastfeeding' on page 43 for more information. You could also express any leftover milk after each feed. Stopping feeding from the affected breast could make the mastitis worse, but if you find breastfeeding too painful you could express milk to feed to your baby from a bottle. Your milk is still safe to feed to your baby and won't pass the infection on to them due to the milk's anti-infective properties.

Other ways to help ease mastitis:

▶ Wear loose clothing and a soft, comfortable bra.

▶ Place a warm flannel on the affected area, or have a warm bath or shower, to help ease the pain and encourage the milk to flow.

▶ Gently stroke the affected area, moving your hand towards your nipple.

▶ Take ibuprofen (or if you prefer, paracetamol) to help relieve the inflammation and ease the pain.

▶ If the mastitis doesn't improve within 24 hours, or your symptoms worsen, see your GP as soon as possible as you may have an infection that will need to be treated with an antibiotic. Warning: left untreated, mastitis can develop into an abscess that will need immediate medical attention[4].

Cluster (frequent) feeding

Cluster feeding is where your baby has several feeds close together – perhaps with only a half an hour gap and sometimes feeds 2 to 3 hours at a time. Your baby can cluster feed at any time of the day or night, but it tends to happen most often in the evening. There could be several reasons for your baby wanting to feed more often and for longer; you may not produce as much milk at night when you're tired; your milk might not be as rich in the evening as is it is during the day; your baby may have slept quite a lot during the day and is now having to catch up on feeding; your baby may just enjoy the calming and soothing effects of nursing, or they may have colic and need the comfort of suckling.

Most babies only cluster feed in the first month or so – but it could go on for a little longer if they are suffering from colic and they could do it again during growth spurts.

Coping with cluster feeding

The best way to cope with cluster feeding is to let your baby feed as often as they want. Avoid supplementing your milk with formula, as this will reduce your milk flow. Remember that your body will produce the right amount of milk for your baby, if you let them feed on demand. Cluster feeds often follow a regular pattern each evening, so if you think a cluster feed is going to happen, you could prepare for it by making sure you have had something to eat and drink beforehand. View cluster feeding as a time to sit down and relax. You could read a book while breastfeeding, phone a friend, or watch TV. But if you need to be on the move you could try breastfeeding your baby while carrying them in a sling to free up your hands; there are slings available that have a breastfeeding position to allow you to do this.

Cluster feeding can be really tiring, especially as it often happens at a time when you want to start winding down and have some time to yourself. Bear in mind this stage will pass, so try to go with the flow if you can. On a positive note, you may find that your baby sleeps for longer during the night during a period of cluster feeding.

Breast refusal

Breast refusal is the completely opposite problem to cluster feeding. This is where your baby fights and struggles when you put them to the breast, which can be stressful and upsetting. They may refuse to feed at all, start sucking and then stop, or appear distressed and unwilling to continue. Or your baby might not refuse the breast, but be very fussy and hard to feed.

Reasons for breast refusal and possible solutions

There are a number of reasons why your baby might not want to feed, even though they appear hungry or it is a while since they were fed.

Your baby is tired due to the birth or the sedative effects of the pain relief you had – this should only be temporary. Keep on offering your baby the breast every hour or two. If the drowsiness and lack of interest in breastfeeding continues beyond a few hours tell your midwife or health visitor.

Your baby has waited too long for a feed – some babies become upset if they aren't fed as soon as they are hungry; try to respond quickly to your baby's early hunger cues, such as opening and closing their mouth, or rooting for the nipple, before they start crying.

Your baby is having problems latching on – check you are holding your baby in the correct position at the breast. See 'Position your baby correctly' on page 43, 'Make sure your baby latches on properly' on page 44 and 'Your baby isn't latching on properly' on page 57. If your breast is engorged, try expressing some milk (into a bottle to store for later); this will make it easier for your baby to latch on.

Your baby has thrush – which is making their mouth sore and feeding painful. You will need to see your GP as soon as possible if you think your baby has thrush. They will be able to prescribe an antifungal treatment to clear it up. In the meantime, you could try a baking soda solution to help relieve the itching and discomfort and encourage your baby to start feeding again. For more information see 'Thrush' on page 153.

Your baby has a blocked nose – making it hard for them to breathe and breastfeed at the same time. You could try to ease the congestion by exposing your baby to a steamy atmosphere. For example run a hot bath or shower, then take your baby in the bathroom to inhale the steam for a few minutes before offering the breast again. Alternatively, use a saline spray or place some saline drops in each nostril just before a feed. These help to thin the mucus and clear the nose. Another option is to use a nasal aspirator to remove the mucus from your baby's nose.

Tip

Note: Vapour rubs are not recommended for babies under three months, but there are vapour oils that can be placed in a vaporiser or bowl of warm water to release oils into your baby's room and are safe to use from birth – for further details see Useful Products, page 194.

Your baby has an ear infection – which means breastfeeding is painful if they are placed on the infected ear. Placing them on your other breast means they won't be pressing on their infected ear, which should make feeding more comfortable.

Your baby is frustrated because they can't get enough milk – this could either be due to your milk not letting down or a lack of milk. It could be that you are feeling tired or stressed from the demands of parenthood and this is affecting your letdown reflex. If you think this is the case, try to relax for a few minutes. Hand your baby to your partner, or a trusted family member or friend and take a break. Put your feet up and watch your favourite TV programme, or listen to some relaxing music. Then try feeding your baby again.

If your letdown reflex is unreliable you can improve it by doing less and relaxing more. For your milk to let down efficiently – especially in the early days – you need to feel relaxed, calm and unhurried before and during each feed. For more tips on how to reduce stress, rest and relax see page 169.

If you think you don't have enough milk you will need to build up your milk supply by resting as much as possible, eating well, drinking whenever you feel thirsty (if your urine is pale you are drinking enough) and feeding your baby more often. Expressing milk in between feeds can also help to stimulate milk production.

In the meantime, if your baby won't settle and all else fails, as a last resort and to avoid your baby going hungry, you could offer them a formula feed. But if you plan to continue breastfeeding, try not to do this very often.

Traditional milk boosters

Fennel or fenugreek tea and porridge oats are traditional remedies for low milk supply; while there is only anecdotal evidence they work, it wouldn't hurt to give them a try. You can make fennel or fenugreek tea by placing two teaspoons of the seeds in a cafetière. Pour on boiling water and replace the cafetière lid. Leave to brew for a few minutes, then press down the plunger and pour. You can also buy teabags containing fennel, fenugreek and other ingredients believed to boost milk supply. See Useful Products, page 194.

More ways to handle breast refusal

Stay calm and avoid trying to force your baby to feed – as this will make them more likely to struggle and fret. If your baby seems upset, focus on pacifying them first; try cuddling, rocking or singing to them, or carry them around the room until they settle down and then try feeding them again.

Try a different feeding position – feed your baby while lying on your side on the settee or bed with your baby alongside you.

Tip

Note: Don't feed your baby in bed or on a sofa if you are feeling tired or have had a drink and could fall asleep, as this raises the risk of your baby suffocating.

Or try the clutch or football position – sit upright with your baby lying down, their legs and feet tucked horizontally under your arm.

Supporting their spine along your arm, cradle their head in your hand with their mouth in line with your nipple.

Try breastfeeding your baby when they are sleepy – some babies who battle with the breast when they are wide-awake feed better when they are drowsy.

Express your milk – and feed it to your baby from a bottle, while still encouraging your baby to breastfeed and trying to find a solution to the problem. Your baby will still benefit from your breast milk and avoid the risk of becoming dehydrated or undernourished, while it will help to prevent you becoming engorged, or developing mastitis.

Seek support

If you are having problems with breastfeeding and are unable to resolve them then speak to your midwife, health visitor or doctor. Alternatively, organisations such as Baby Café, Milk Matters, National Childbirth Trust, The Breastfeeding Network and La Leche League all have trained breastfeeding counsellors who can offer you support and advice. For more information see the Directory, page 198.

If you decide to stop breastfeeding

Breastfeeding isn't for everyone so don't feel guilty if you decide to stop. However make absolutely sure that it is the right decision for you, as some mums spend months regretting stopping and wondering if they gave up too easily. It's difficult to restart breastfeeding once your milk supply has dwindled.

Once you have made the decision, gradually replace breastfeeds with formula feeds over a couple of weeks to avoid your breasts becoming engorged, and to help your baby adjust to the change. If you want to stop straight away you will need to express milk to prevent engorgement, until your milk supply gradually reduces.

How to combine breast and bottle-feeding

Mixed feeding, which involves combining breast and formula feeding, is another alternative to stopping breastfeeding completely. It can help to ease the pressure if you are finding breastfeeding tough, while your baby will still enjoy the benefits of your breast milk. You can choose which feeds you want to replace with formula. For example, if you find you have less milk last thing at night when you are tired, you could use formula then. Or if you like to pop out during the day, you could give your baby a bottle of formula instead of a breastfeed. Bear in mind that the less often you feed your baby the less milk you'll produce. That said, many mums find that combining breast and formula feeding is a compromise that works for them.

Real-life experiences of two breastfeeding mums

The secret of successful breastfeeding is to tailor how you do it to suit the needs of both you and your baby. Here are two real-life stories from breastfeeding mums that show how they made it work for them.

Andrea, 33 – first-time mum to Kieran

Andrea found that feeding Kieran expressed breast milk from a bottle during the day and nursing him at the breast during the night enabled her to get out and about more easily.

She explained: 'Breastfeeding made me feel isolated in the first few weeks. Kieran fed almost every half an hour. One of the main problems I found was a lack of places to breastfeed in private when out and about. Even at home I found it a problem if we had visitors and Kieran needed a feed, as I didn't like feeding in front of most people, so I had to go in a bedroom and miss out on the conversation. The same thing happened if I visited friends or family. It started to get me down, so after the first two weeks I started expressing my milk and feeding him from a bottle. This meant I could go out during the day and feed Kieran without having to worry about being in the right place at the right time to feed him; I still fed him on the breast at night, as it was easier than having to fumble around with bottles. This worked well for me and it enabled me to feed Kieran entirely on breast milk for the first six months. I think it's important to realise that not all babies want to be fed the same way. After the first few weeks I found that Kieran didn't like me holding him in my arms to feed him – he actually preferred to lie on the floor or bed with me lying alongside him.'

Stacey, 30 – first-time mum to Mila

Stacey found that combining breast and bottle-feeding helped to prevent her baby suffering from wind and gave her some 'me-time'.

She told me: 'I breastfed Mila exclusively until she was about eight weeks old, then I did a combination of breast and formula.

By three months I was expressing one bottle of milk to feed her during the day and then feeding her from the breast through the night, the rest of the time I gave her formula milk.

'Mila was born four weeks early weighing only 4 lb 11 oz (2.126 kg); within five days she weighed 5 lb 3 oz (2.353 kg), which reassured me that by breastfeeding I was doing the best I could for her. I had a real sense of achievement seeing Mila's weight increase week on week. The closeness you feel being able to feed your baby and knowing only you can do it is amazing.

'As she was small she fed often, which was very demanding. I was especially sleep deprived because I had been in hospital the week before the birth and hadn't had much opportunity to sleep. The decision to breastfeed means that although everyone can do everything else, you are the one that needs to feed your baby and therefore broken sleep is the best you are going to get and it's hard!

'After a few weeks Mila seemed to be in a lot of pain during and after feeding and it was difficult to get her wind up. It wasn't colic but using Infacol helped a little. Then I noticed that when she drank my expressed milk from a bottle the wind was nowhere near as bad. People say breastfed babies don't get wind – this is untrue because mine did. I carried on feeding her expressed milk from a bottle for around eight weeks, but in the end I felt it was making twice the work for me and as Mila was clearly in pain after feeding I made the decision to introduce formula. It was hard, as I really enjoyed breastfeeding and I knew she was thriving, but I didn't want her to be in pain. Carrying on as I was also got me down, as I had little sleep and couldn't go very far without her needing to feed and I didn't want to be in the house all day. Once I introduced formula it meant that my partner and family could help with feeds, so I could have more sleep and a bit of "me time". It also meant that I dared go out for the day without the fear of how and where I was going to feed her. I don't regret my decision at all as I think it was best for both of us.

'I always said I wouldn't give myself a hard time if I couldn't breastfeed but I did! Once you stop breastfeeding as often, your milk supply drops; every time this happened I kept "upping the ante" to get my supply back. Even now when I'm close to giving in completely I think "come on you can pull this back" and I do. When I was struggling I felt like nobody understood – I had friends that had managed to breastfeed easily, so I didn't think they would understand and I thought those who formula fed would think, why bother? But after talking to other mums I realised they felt the same and could relate to how I felt.'

Hopefully these examples have given you some insight into the kind of issues you might face when breastfeeding, as well as some ideas on how to resolve them.

Bottle-feeding pros and cons

Pros

Other people, such as your partner and family can feed your baby – so you can have a break, which can be beneficial – especially if you are suffering from postnatal illness (PNI, formerly known as postnatal depression). It also gives your partner the opportunity to bond with their baby.

Bottle-feeding your baby allows you to focus on them – without having to worry about whether you are feeding them correctly, or if they are getting enough milk; you can see how much milk your baby is getting, which can be reassuring.

Breastfeeding can be a little uncomfortable at first – bottle-feeding is not.

Cons

Formula has to be bought – and can be expensive.

Bottles have to be washed and sterilised and formula has to be mixed – which is time-consuming.

Formula is not identical to breast milk – though most now contain prebiotics, probiotics and essential fatty acids, they don't provide all of the health benefits breast milk does.

You might not feel the unique bond you would have if you were breastfeeding – because anyone can bottle-feed your baby.

Once you have made the decision to bottle-feed you will need to know about the different types of formula, how to sterilise the feeding equipment, how to mix a bottle of formula and how to give your baby a bottle.

Types of infant formula

Most infant formulas are made from cow's milk, which contains more protein and fewer sugars than breast milk, so it has to be modified to make it suitable for babies. You can also buy formulas based on goat's milk, hydrolysed protein, or soya, all of which are modified to resemble breast milk.

For the first six months of their life your baby should be fed a type of formula known as 'first milk', which usually contains more whey protein than casein, making it easier to digest than casein-based follow-on milks.

Goat's milk based formula is claimed to be more easily digested than cow's milk based formula, but is much more expensive.

Hydrolysed formulas are suitable for babies with a cow's milk allergy or intolerance. Cow's milk *allergy* (CMA) involves the body's immune system reacting to the protein in cow's milk. Symptoms can include eczema, skin rashes, hives, vomiting, diarrhoea, colic and, in severe cases, difficulty breathing. Cow's milk *intolerance* doesn't involve the immune system and is due to an inability to digest lactose (milk sugar) in milk. Signs of intolerance are less severe than CMA and can include diarrhoea, bloating and wind. If you suspect your baby has a cow's milk allergy or intolerance, see your doctor or health visitor before giving your baby a different type of formula. If your doctor believes your baby is allergic to cow's milk they may prescribe a fully hydrolysed-protein formula. If they think your baby has a milk intolerance they may prescribe a fully hydrolysed formula or recommend that you buy a lactose-free formula instead.

Hydrolysed formulas still contain cow's milk, but the milk protein and milk sugar has been broken down so that babies can digest it more easily and are less likely to react to it. Fully hydrolysed formula is also lactose free so it is suitable for babies with CMA or lactose intolerance and is available on prescription.

Partially hydrolysed whey formula is made from whey protein and is claimed to be more easily digested than casein-protein-based formulas and therefore helpful for babies who suffer from wind or colic.

Soya-based formula is made from soya beans. It is also designed for babies with lactose (milk sugar) intolerance or cow's milk protein allergy, but quite often a baby that can't tolerate cow's milk can't tolerate soya-based formula either. Soya-based formula isn't usually recommended for babies under six months of age because it contains plant oestrogens and should only be given to your baby on the advice of your GP, health visitor or paediatrician.

Other added ingredients can include vitamins and minerals, vegetable oils, fish oils, and prebiotics in the form of sugars called oligosaccharides, that promote the growth of 'good' bacteria in your baby's gut. All infant formulas have to meet regulations to ensure they are safe to give to babies. However, there are still slight differences in the composition of different brands, so if one seems to disagree with your baby you could try another one. Formula is sold ready-made in cartons and in powder form ready to be mixed with water; cartons work out a lot more expensive, but are more convenient for days out or when you are on holiday

How to sterilise feeding equipment

All bottles, including teats, retaining rings, caps, tongs and milk scoops must be washed in hot soapy water, rinsed and then sterilised before each use. This is to kill off any bacteria, viruses and fungi that could collect and make your baby ill. You can use the dishwasher to clean them, or wash them by hand in hot soapy water, using a bottlebrush to get the bottles thoroughly clean. Clean the inside of the teats as well as the outside by turning them inside out. Throw away any damaged teats or badly scratched bottles, as these can harbour bacteria.

You can then sterilise the equipment using an electric steam or microwave steriliser, by microwaving or boiling, or with a cold-water steriliser. To keep everything sterile leave the sterilised items in the steriliser with the lid on and only remove a bottle as and when you need to make a feed up. Clean and disinfect the work surface you're going to use first[5]. Always wash your hands before handling sterilised equipment. Use sterilised tongs to remove the teat, lid, retaining ring, and cap from the steriliser to avoid contaminating the remaining items.

Electric steam sterilising

Electric steam sterilisers are fast, efficient and easy to use. They can sterilise equipment in as little as 6 minutes plus time for cooling. They can keep bottles sterilised for up to 24 hours if you don't lift the lid. Most steam sterilisers hold up to six bottles and have a rack for smaller items like teats and dummies. Place items with the openings face down to make sure the steam gets inside them. Always check that equipment is suitable for steaming, as some items, such as breast pump parts, may not be.

Microwave steamers

Microwave steamers take as little as 2 minutes to work, plus time for cooling. The contents stay sterile for up to 24 hours if you keep the steriliser closed[6].

Microwaving

You can also buy feeding bottles that can be sterilised in the microwave without a steamer. Fill the bottle halfway with water and place it upright inside the microwave, without the teat, cap or cover on, to prevent pressure building up inside; immerse these in water in a microwave-safe container. Place the container next to the bottle and microwave everything on full power for 90 seconds.

Boiling

If your baby's bottles are suitable you can sterilise them by boiling – though it is less convenient than more modern methods. Use a large pan with a lid; if possible use a new pan and keep it just for sterilising. Fill the pan with water completely covering the feeding equipment. Check there are no air bubbles inside the bottles and teats, then cover the pan and boil for at least 10 minutes[7]. If you're not using the bottles immediately, assemble them fully with the teat and lid in place to prevent the inside of the sterilised bottle and the inside and outside of the teat being contaminated. If you use this method often inspect the teats regularly, as boiling can damage them quicker than other sterilising methods[8].

Cold-water sterilising

This method involves sterilising equipment with a solution of sodium hypochlorite made by adding cold water to sterilising fluid or tablets. Follow the manufacturer's instructions on the pack carefully. You can buy a cold-water sterilising unit that has a weighted grid to keep equipment submerged. Alternatively you could use a clean plastic container or bucket with a lid, with a plate to keep the items beneath the solution.

When you put the bottles and teats in the solution check there are no pockets of trapped air in them. Leave the feeding equipment in for at least the required amount of time (usually 15 to 30 minutes). Leave items in the solution until you are about to use them – they will stay sterile for 24 hours. Items can be added and removed from the same solution throughout that time, but you must change the solution every 24 hours. Shake each item as you get it out to remove excess solution. Depending on the brand you use you may want to rinse them with cool, boiled water before using[9].

How to mix a bottle of formula

When preparing a bottle of formula follow the instructions on the pack carefully. It's vitally important that the milk is made up accurately. If you add too little milk powder your baby may fail to thrive. If you add too much, your baby may become constipated or dehydrated. Below are basic instructions for making up a bottle.

1. Boil some tap water and leave it to cool in the kettle for no more than half an hour[10] to ensure it remains at a temperature of at least 70˚C, to kill any harmful bacteria.

2. Clean and disinfect the surface you are going to use. Wash your hands thoroughly.

3. Measure the exact amount of water required into a sterilised bottle.

4. Loosely fill the scoop with formula. Level it off using the flat edge of a clean, dry knife or the leveller provided. Add the correct number of scoops to the bottle.

5. Place the teat on the bottle. Screw on the retaining ring and cover the teat with the cap.

6. Shake the bottle until the powder is completely dissolved.

7. Hold the bottle under a cold tap to cool it until it is lukewarm.

Preparing feeds in advance

Ideally you should make up each bottle as you need it, to avoid the risk of bacteria infecting the milk. Powdered formulas can contain bacteria that can multiply once made up, especially if they are kept at room temperature.

However, there will be times when making a bottle from scratch isn't convenient – for example in the middle of the night, or when you are out and about. The World Health Organization (WHO) says you can safely make bottles up in advance, so long as you cool each bottle quickly, by holding them under a cold tap and store them in the fridge at no higher than 5 °C, for no longer than 24 hours. Reheat in a container of warm water for no longer than 15 minutes. Never reheat a feed in a microwave, as the milk may heat unevenly and burn your baby's mouth and throat.

Alternatively, keep the boiled water in a washed and scalded Thermos flask and pre-measure the correct amount of formula into a sterilised airtight container. Make up the formula in a sterilised bottle as and when needed. By using water that is hotter than 70 °C you will kill off unwanted bacteria and when you cool it down you will slow down bacteria growth. If you are going out with your baby, take the cold feeds out of the fridge just before you leave and put them in a cool bag with ice packs. Reheat as needed.

How to give your baby a bottle

1. Find a comfortable place to sit.

2. Hold your baby fairly upright in your bent arm, so their head and neck are well supported and they can make eye contact with you.

3. With your other hand hold the bottle slightly tilted, so the teat is always full of milk and so your baby is less likely to take in air.

4. Gently touch your baby's cheek with the teat to encourage them to root for the teat and start sucking.

5. If your baby stops feeding or seems unsettled then stop for a burping break (see below).

6. Let your baby decide when they've had enough milk – don't try to force them to finish the bottle.

7. Never leave your baby to feed on their own with a propped-up bottle, as they could choke.

8. Once a bottle of formula or breast milk has been drunk from, you must throw away any unused milk within one hour. Untouched formula or defrosted breast milk kept out at room temperature should be discarded within 2 hours. Untouched

freshly expressed milk will keep for up to 6 hours at room temperature (no more than 25°C). Never reheat a feed, as bacteria flourish in warm milk.

Bottle-feeding dos and don'ts

Do feed on demand. This could be every couple of hours for the first few weeks. As your baby grows they'll be able to take more milk and go for longer in between feeds.

Don't re-boil previously boiled water, as this changes the mineral content of the water – always fill the kettle with fresh water.

Don't warm a bottle in the microwave, as they can cause hot spots in the milk that could scald your baby's mouth. Warm in a container of warm water or use an electric bottle warmer according to the instructions.

Do double-check the temperature of the milk by dripping a small amount on the inside of your wrist. It should feel lukewarm not hot.

Feeding guide

As a rough guide, per day your baby will need 150 ml to 200 ml of formula for each kilogramme they weigh[11]. So, if your baby weighs 6 lb 10 oz (3 kg), they'll need 450 ml to 600 ml of formula in 24 hours. However all babies have individual needs, so it's best to give them as much as they want. Babies usually know when they have had enough!

How to burp your baby

Whether breastfed or bottle-fed, most babies swallow air during a feed, which can make them uncomfortable and cause colic or lead to them bringing up some of their feed. Breastfed babies usually swallow less air during feeds than bottle-fed babies – though if you have a lot of milk that flows quickly your baby may gulp it down faster and ingest more air.

If you are bottle-feeding formula or expressed breast milk, you can help to reduce the amount of air your baby swallows by buying anti-colic bottles and teats – for more information on bottle-feeding equipment see page 22; and 'Colic' on page 134. Sitting your baby up when they are feeding from a bottle could also help.

With experience you'll recognise when your baby needs burping – they will usually show their discomfort by pulling away from the bottle or breast, crying and squirming. It's also a good idea to burp your baby when you change sides during breastfeeding or halfway through bottle-feeding.

Below are three ways to burp a baby – you could try each one and see which method works best for your baby. As your baby gets older you should find they need less burping, as they tend to swallow less air. Your baby may bring up a little milk along with the trapped air, so it's a good idea to have a muslin cloth strategically placed on your lap or shoulder.

1. **Sitting your baby on your knee** – lean them slightly forwards, with the palm of one hand on their upper chest to support their body and your fingers gently cupping their chin and jaw. Using your other hand gently rub or pat their back. The

upright position encourages the air bubbles to release from the stomach.

2. **Holding your baby upright against you** – with their chin resting on your shoulder. Using one hand to support their head and shoulders, gently rub or pat their back with your other hand.

3. **Placing your baby face down across your lap** – so their tummy is on one of your legs and their head is on the other, turned to the side. The weight of your baby's body puts gentle pressure on their tummy, helping them to bring up any trapped air. You can gently rub or pat their back to help the process along.

If none of these methods work, you could try giving your baby a gentle tummy massage – see 'Cut crying with massage' on page 115. Or, if trapped wind becomes a problem, you could try using over-the-counter oral drops that contain a substance called simethicone, which helps to break down the trapped wind so it's easier for your baby to burp up – see also 'Colic' on page 134.

CHAPTER 3

CARE FOR YOUR BABY

When you first become parents you will find that you need to master a lot of new skills very quickly in order to care for your new baby. You may have attended antenatal classes through the NHS, National Childbirth Trust, or another private provider and have picked up a few of the basics. However, if like me you find changing a nappy, bathing and dressing a live and kicking baby is rather different to practising on a baby doll, or watching a demonstration by an NCT teacher or midwife, you should find this chapter useful. Of course the best way to learn is by doing and you will probably find you develop your own ways of doing things based on what works best for you and your baby, but in the early days it helps if you have a few pointers that you can refer to.

In this chapter:

▶ How to pick up and hold your baby safely
▶ Changing your baby's nappy
▶ Understand your baby's poo – what's normal
▶ … And what's not
▶ How to bath your baby
▶ 'Top and tail' your baby
▶ Caring for the umbilical stump

- ▶ Cutting your baby's nails
- ▶ Give your baby regular 'tummy time'
- ▶ How to dress and undress your baby
- ▶ Keep your baby at the right temperature
- ▶ Getting out and about with your baby
- ▶ Going on holiday with your baby

How to pick up and hold your baby

Many new parents feel a bit frightened of handling their newborn because they seem so fragile. Your baby does need gentle and careful handling but there is no need to worry – your baby is far more resilient than you think.

Move slowly and smoothly when lifting and holding your baby – avoid sudden jerky movements, as this may startle them. Remember your baby is used to feeling safe and secure in the womb.

Your baby is unable to support their own head, so always do it for them. To pick your baby up, slide one hand under their head and one under their bottom. Use a forearm to give extra support to their spine, before lifting them slowly towards you.

To hold your baby, cradle their head in the crook of your bent elbow, using your forearm to support their body. As they get bigger, you may need to use both arms.

You can also hold your baby upright against your chest with one hand supporting their bottom and the other one cradling their head and neck. Once your baby is able to hold their head up they will probably prefer to be held in this position, as they will be able to see more of what is going on around them.

Changing your baby's nappy

If you practised putting a nappy on a doll at antenatal classes you may have thought it was pretty straightforward. However, when faced with a wriggling baby you may find it is a little trickier than you thought.

1. Make sure you have everything you will need close to hand. A lot of new babies cry when they are having their nappy changed and it's easy to get into a flap, if you have to start looking around for things. So grab the essentials – a changing mat or a clean towel, a clean nappy, a nappy liner (if used), a nappy sack to hold the soiled nappy or nappy liner, cotton wool and tepid water or baby wipes, and a barrier cream such as petroleum jelly or zinc and castor oil cream, etc. You may also need a change of clothing for your baby.

2. Place the changing mat/towel on a flat, stable surface and lie your baby down on it.

3. Open the tabs on the dirty nappy and fold them over so they don't stick to your baby.

4. Pull down the front of the dirty nappy. If your baby has pooed, use the front part of the nappy to wipe your baby's bottom from front to back.

5. Now gently grasp your baby's ankles and raise their bottom to lift them off the changing mat enough to allow you to fold the dirty nappy in half with the clean outer part facing upwards. Lower your baby back onto the nappy.

6. Clean your baby's bottom thoroughly using wipes or cotton wool and water. If your baby is a girl wipe from front to back, to avoid bacterial infection. If you have a baby boy gently clean around his testicles (balls) and penis, but don't try to pull the foreskin back, as it will still be attached to the penis and could tear. Check skin folds and crevices for any hidden poo.

7. Open the clean nappy and raise your baby's bottom off the mat again to remove the dirty nappy and position out of your baby's reach and place the back half of the clean nappy under your baby's bottom.

8. Apply a barrier cream such as petroleum jelly, or a nappy rash cream such as zinc and castor oil over the whole of the nappy area. Fasten the nappy, making sure it is not too tight.

Understand your baby's poo – what's normal

Your newborn will pass meconium for the first couple of days after the birth. Meconium is a greenish-black colour and has a sticky consistency. It is made up of the amniotic fluid your baby swallowed while they were in your womb, and the substances the amniotic fluid contains, such as mucus and skin cells.

If you breastfeed your baby

By about the third day your baby's poo will change to a mustardy yellow colour. It will have a fairly runny, but grainy texture and a mild, sweetish smell, because breast milk is well digested and produces very little waste. For the first few weeks they may poo during or after every feed. This will eventually settle down to a regular pattern where your baby may poo at the same time each day, or poo once every few days; so long as their poo is soft and easily passed, this is fine.

If you formula-feed your baby

If you formula-feed your baby their poo will be a pale yellow or brownish-yellow colour. It will be quite thick – a bit like the consistency of toothpaste, and will have a fairly strong smell – because formula milk is not as well digested as breast milk. Formula-fed babies are more likely to become constipated – for details of how you can relieve it, see 'Constipation' on page 138.

If you change from breastfeeding to formula feeding

Your baby's poo will gradually change to the colour and texture described above. Try to make the changeover gradual, to help your baby adjust to the new milk and reduce the risk of them becoming constipated; however if you decide to stop breastfeeding quickly, offering your baby extra boiled water will help prevent constipation.

... and what's not

Very runny, more frequent poos – this may mean they have diarrhoea. Breastfed babies are less likely to suffer from diarrhoea because breast milk contains probiotics (good bacteria) and prebiotics, which promote the growth of good bacteria in their gut. See also 'Diarrhoea' on page 144.

Small, dry, pellet-like poos or large hard poos – usually mean your baby is constipated. Formula-fed babies are more likely to suffer from constipation than breastfed babies, because formula milk is harder to digest. Using too much formula when making up a bottle can cause constipation, so if your baby has constipation check that you are mixing the milk correctly. Another cause could be dehydration in hot weather. See also 'Constipation' on page 138.

Green poo – if you are breastfeeding this could be due to your baby getting too much lactose (milk sugar). This can happen if your baby feeds frequently because they are only getting the foremilk but not the rich, filling hindmilk at the end of the feed – hence they are taking in more sugar. To correct this make sure your baby empties the first breast before putting them on the other. If your baby is bottle-fed it could be the brand of formula you are using that is making your baby's poo dark green[12]. It may be worth changing to a different brand to see if that helps. If that makes no difference speak to your health visitor or GP.

Very pale poo – can be due to jaundice, which is common in newborns. Jaundice makes your newborn's skin and the whites of their eyes look yellow. It generally clears up by the time your baby is about two weeks. Talk to your midwife, health visitor or doctor if you think your baby has jaundice.

Chalky white poos – if your baby passes these tell your midwife, health visitor, or doctor, as it could mean they have liver problems, especially if they have had jaundice for more than two weeks.

How to bath your baby

Bathing your baby can seem a little daunting in the beginning, but once you have done it a few times it will become automatic. Some babies love being in the water, while others are less keen and make sure you know it! It is down to you how often you bath your baby. In the first few weeks a bath three times a week is enough, if you 'top and tail' them in between bath times i.e. wash their face, hands, genitals and bottom (see below). If your baby has eczema you will find information on bathing and caring for their skin on page 147. Below are some basic steps you can follow to make bath time as trouble-free as possible[13].

1. Choose a time when you can bath your baby without being interrupted. It is best to bath them in between feeds, so they are content and less likely to bring up a feed. If your baby seems to find a bath relaxing it might be a good idea to bath them in the evening to form the beginning of a bedtime routine.

Tip

Safety note: Never leave your baby unattended, or turn away from your baby, when they are in the bath. If the phone rings, or someone knocks on your door and you need to answer it, *always* pick your baby up and take them with you.

2. Choose the place you find easiest – this could be a plastic baby bath in the warmth of the living room, or the family bath, with a

bath support, a baby bath that attaches to it, or a bucket bath; for the first few weeks I bathed my daughter in the washbasin in the bathroom, because it was quick and easy! Make sure the room is warm enough. Close doors and windows to avoid draughts.

3. Gather together everything you'll need:
   - ▶ A baby bath (if you are using one)
   - ▶ Cotton wool balls
   - ▶ A clean flannel or a sponge
   - ▶ A bath thermometer, if you have one, for checking the water temperature – though you could use your elbow
   - ▶ Baby liquid cleanser, if used
   - ▶ Baby shampoo, if used
   - ▶ Baby lotion or oil – if your baby has dry skin
   - ▶ A changing mat
   - ▶ A clean small towel or baby towel – hooded towels are great for wrapping your baby in from head to toe
   - ▶ A clean nappy, nappy liner (if used) and nappy sack
   - ▶ Clean clothing

4. Place the towel next to the changing mat and lie your baby down on it.

5. Fill the bath. If you are using a baby cleanser pour a little in first before adding cold water first then hot until it is a depth of about 13 cm and at the right temperature. If you have a bath thermometer it should read no higher than 37 °C to 38 °C. If you use your elbow the bath should feel lukewarm. If you are using a baby bath, place it next to your baby.

6. Undress your baby. If they have pooed their nappy, clean their bottom and genital area with cotton wool and water.

7. Wash your baby's face and hair. Wrap them in the towel and hold them over the bath securely with one arm supporting their head, neck and body. Use your other hand to gently clean their face using cotton wool or a flannel moistened in the bath water. You may notice some tiny white spots, known as milk spots, or milia, on your baby's face; these are caused by your baby's developing sweat glands and are harmless.

    Next wet your baby's scalp, apply baby shampoo or a liquid cleanser if used, and massage gently before rinsing. You will notice two soft spots (fontanelles) on your baby's head where the skull has not yet fully closed – one on the top and one at the back of the head. It is perfectly safe to gently touch and wash these areas.

8. Lower your baby gently into the bath with one arm supporting their head and neck and your hand holding their arms and your other hand supporting their bottom.

9. Continue to support their head and neck with one arm and use your other hand to wash them down with a sponge or flannel.

10. Lift your baby out of the bath, and lie them down on the towel. Wrap them up and gently blot them dry. Lie your baby down on the changing mat. Let them have a kick around for a minute or two to allow the air to get to the areas that are normally covered with a nappy.

11. Gently massage in baby lotion or baby oil, if used.

12. Put your baby's nappy and clothing on.

'Top and tail' your baby

1. Check the room is warm enough.

2. Gather together everything you'll need:

   ▶ A small bowl
   ▶ Cotton wool balls or pads
   ▶ A clean flannel or sponge
   ▶ Baby cleanser or baby wipes
   ▶ A changing mat
   ▶ A clean towel
   ▶ A clean nappy, nappy liner (if used) and nappy sack
   ▶ Clean clothes

3. Fill the small bowl with lukewarm water and check it with your elbow or use a thermometer – the temperature should be no higher than 37 °C to 38 °C – it should feel lukewarm.

4. Place the towel on the changing mat. Lie your baby down on top of the towel and changing mat and undress them.

5. 'Top' your baby; using dampened cotton wool gently wipe your baby's eyes from the inner to outer corners. Use fresh cotton wool for each eye to avoid spreading infection. Use fresh cotton wool to wipe inside the outer parts of the ears and behind them. Don't clean inside your baby's ear canals, as you could damage their eardrums. Use fresh moistened cotton wool to clean your baby's face, neck and hands.

6. 'Tail' your baby; with a fresh piece of dampened cotton wool clean their bottom and genital area remembering to wipe front

to back for girls; if they have pooed use a mild baby cleanser or baby wipe.

Caring for the umbilical cord stump

When one new mum, Emma, told me: 'I didn't have a clue what to do about the cord stump,' she was echoing how many new parents feel. Even though the cord stump can look a bit unpleasant, it's nothing to worry about.

During your pregnancy the umbilical cord provides nutrients and oxygen to your developing baby. After your baby's birth the umbilical cord isn't needed – so it's clamped in two places with plastic clips and cut to leave a stump around 2 to 3 cm long; there are no nerves in the cord, so your baby won't feel anything. Some midwives remove the remaining clamp after a few days, while others leave it on until the stump shrivels up and falls off – usually about seven days after the birth. Until this happens, and the belly button is completely healed, you need to make sure that the area is kept clean and dry, to avoid infection.

You can clean your baby's stump with plain water, or with a mild, liquid baby cleanser added to the bathwater. Gently blot the stump dry with a clean, soft towel. Make sure it is completely dry before putting a nappy on. You don't need to use an antiseptic on the stump, so long as you keep it clean. To help prevent wee or poo getting on the stump and allow air to circulate around the wound fold down the waist of your baby's nappy when you put it on. If the stump does get wee or poo on it wash it off thoroughly as soon as possible. Your baby's belly button will probably be completely healed by about seven to ten days after the stump falls off. If the area looks reddened, or smells unpleasant, ask your midwife, health visitor or GP to check it in case it's the start of an infection.

Dealing with peeling skin

While your baby was in the womb a white, waxy coating called vernix protected their skin. Once they are born and their skin is exposed to the air and the vernix is washed off, the top layer of skin dries out – hence the peeling. The skin on the whole of their body may peel, but it tends to be more noticeable on the hands and feet. This should settle down in a week or two, but in the meantime you could try massaging a small amount of baby oil into the affected areas.

Cutting your baby's nails

It's best to keep your baby's nails short, so they are less likely to scratch themselves. Avoid cutting your baby's nails until they are at least four weeks old, as newborn babies' nails are very soft and it can be hard to tell what is nail and what is skin. If scratching becomes a problem you could put scratch mittens on their hands. After about a month your baby's nails should be hard enough for you to trim them. Use baby nail scissors with rounded edges to avoid the risk of nicking their skin. You may find it easier to trim them while your baby is asleep. Another option is to gently file them using an emery board.

Give your baby regular 'tummy time'

When I had my children we were advised to place them on their front to go to sleep. But the advice has changed over recent years since research showed that placing your baby on their back to go to sleep reduces the risk of sudden infant death syndrome (SIDS) – formerly known as cot death. However, your baby will benefit from regular, supervised time on their tummy; tummy time makes it easier for them to start moving their body, which will strengthen their neck, shoulders and back and allow them to hold their arms and legs in different positions. Week by week tummy time will encourage your baby to develop their motor skills until they eventually learn to crawl.

Safety first

Always stay with your baby during tummy time. *Never* place your baby on their tummy while they are asleep[14]. Putting a baby down to sleep on their tummy has been shown to increase a baby's risk of SIDS. SIDS is the sudden, unexpected and unexplained death of a seemingly well baby. Fortunately it is rare; around 1 in 3,000 babies a year die from SIDS in the UK. Premature or low birth weight babies are most at risk, and it happens more often in boys. Overheating or being too cold is also thought to increase the risk. Other risk factors include exposure to cigarette smoke, and an unsafe sleeping position – placing them on their back has been shown to be the safest. Other causes include suffocation due to their face being covered by bedding, or becoming trapped between cot slats, or the mattress and the wall. You will find safety rules that help to reduce the risk of SIDS throughout this book (see especially pages 98, 114 and 125).

Another reason to give your baby regular tummy time is that it helps to counteract the flattening effects to the back of the head of lying on their back for a long time. It also gives your baby a different view of the world around them, helping to prevent boredom.

You can start by giving your baby just a couple of minutes tummy time a couple of times a day and then gradually increase the amount of time they spend on their front as they get older. At first you may want to get your baby used to lying on their front by just letting them lie on your chest, or across your knee. Then you can progress to placing them on the floor.

Choose a time when your baby is awake, content and alert. Avoid putting your baby on their front straight after a feed – especially if they suffer from reflux, a condition where they regularly bring up milk (see page 155). A good time might be after a nap or you could incorporate it into your daily routine – for example, you could turn your baby over onto their tummy for a couple of minutes when you change their nappy. You could leave their nappy off at the same time, to allow some air to their bottom; just place a towel or opened nappy beneath them in case they poo or wee.

Make sure the room is warm and remove any pets. Place a blanket on the floor and then lie your baby down on their front on it.

In the beginning your baby will tend to bear a lot of their weight on their face and upper body. As your baby gets stronger they will be able to look around them, which will help them to develop their coordination and their ability to follow objects with their eyes. At around three months your baby will be able to hold their head up and push up on their arms, which will gradually lead on to learning to crawl. Holding a colourful toy above them will encourage them to raise their head and lift themselves up on their forearms in an attempt to reach it. For more information on your baby's development see page 163.

How to dress and undress your baby

Dressing and undressing your baby can seem daunting at first, especially as they are likely to cry because they feel insecure without the comfort and warmth of their clothes. Try not to get flustered – do everything slowly and methodically until you get the hang of it. Start by putting your baby on a changing mat, so that you have both hands free to dress or undress them.

Putting on and taking off a vest

To put a vest on, bunch it up in your hands and open the neck wide. Ease it over your baby's head. Next scrunch up the vest, stretch open one armhole and gently ease your baby's arm through. Repeat with your baby's other arm. Next pull the vest down over your baby's body and fasten the poppers between their legs.

To take a vest off, unfasten the poppers between the legs, lift your baby by gently grasping their ankles and pull the vest up to their armpits. Next guide each arm through the armholes. Open the neck wide and gently pull the vest over your baby's head, keeping it clear of their face.

Putting on and taking off an all-in-one (babygrow)

Put the opened babygrow on the changing mat and lie your baby down on top of it. Concertina one sleeve up and gently ease their hand and arm through. Repeat on the other side. Next place each foot into the feet of the babygrow then fasten the poppers on the legs and body.

To take a babygrow off, undo the poppers and gently lift each leg out. Next gently pull one sleeve by the cuff as you guide the arm out. Repeat with the other sleeve. Use one hand to raise your baby slightly and the other to ease the babygrow from underneath them.

Keep your baby at the right temperature

Your baby can't regulate their body temperature as efficiently as you and, as we've already mentioned, being too hot or too cold are risk factors for SIDS, so it's important to make sure your baby is always at the right temperature; the normal temperature range for a baby is between 36.6°C to 37.2°C. Signs that your baby may be too hot include:

▶ Sweating

▶ Damp hair

▶ Flushed face

▶ Heat rash

▶ Rapid breathing

▶ Fretfulness

▶ Fever

Below are some basic tips on keeping your baby at the right temperature:

▶ Check whether your baby is too hot or too cold by feeling their neck or tummy – not their hands and feet, as they tend to feel cooler than the rest of their body.

▶ If your baby seems too hot, cool them down by removing an item of clothing or blanket.

▶ If your baby's hands or feet feel especially cold indoors and the room is at the right temperature, add an extra layer of clothing or bedding. For outdoors add a hat and mittens, and socks or bootees.

▶ The room your baby sleeps in should be between 16˚C to 20˚C.Check the central heating thermostat, or use a room thermometer to keep an eye on the temperature.

▶ Never put your baby's Moses basket, pram (buggy) or cot next to a radiator, heater or fire, or in direct sunlight and never use a hot water bottle or an electric blanket to warm your baby's bed.

▶ Always place your baby with their feet at the foot of their Moses basket or cot, so they can't slide down under the bedding. Make sure their head stays uncovered by tucking the bedding in no higher than their shoulders. If you use a sleeping bag make sure it is the right size, so your baby can't slip down inside.

▶ Your baby needs to be warmly dressed, especially when they go outside. As a rough guide during the day your baby should wear the same amount of clothes as you are wearing, plus an extra layer, such as a vest or cardigan, depending on the time of year.

▶ Always remove your baby's hat and any extra layers of clothing as soon as you come inside after being outdoors, or if you get into a warm car, bus or train, even if they are asleep and they might wake up, otherwise they could quickly overheat.

▶ Watch out for your baby overheating in the car. If you're on your own with your baby in the car, stop regularly to check they are the right temperature.

▶ Always make sure the room is warm and all doors and windows are shut before changing or bathing your baby.

Getting out and about with your baby

When you're going out with your baby you'll need to be prepared for feeds and nappy changes. Here is a basic checklist of what you'll need to pack either in a large bag or a baby-changing bag when you go out in the first three months.

1. A spare nappy for every couple of hours you plan to be out for.

2. Nappy liners if using reusable nappies.

3. Nappy sacks for used disposable nappies or nappy liners.

4. Gentle baby wipes if used, or a few dampened cotton wool balls in cling film or a sandwich bag.

5. A spare set of clothes in case of nappy leakages, or your baby is sick on their clothing.

6. Bibs to catch the drips if your baby will be feeding from a bottle.

7. One bottle of formula (or expressed) milk, or carton of ready-made baby milk and sterilised bottle, for every couple of hours you expect to be out.

8. A thermal bottle holder to keep your baby's feed cool and prevent bacteria growth.

9. A dummy, if used (see page 111 for more advice about dummies).

10. A changing mat, although some baby changing bags come with an integral changing mat, or you can buy travel changing mats with pouches for nappies and wipes, or ones that fold down small and fit into the changing bag.

11. An extra blanket, if it's cold.

12. A sun hat, if it's hot or sunny.

13. Muslin squares for mopping up sick or spills, or preserving your modesty when breastfeeding.

14. A pain reliever such as Calpol, which comes with a dosage syringe.

Keep your baby safe in the sun

You shouldn't expose your baby to direct sunlight until they are six months old, as their skin doesn't produce enough melanin, the skin pigment that helps to protect the skin from the sun. Also, it is not known how effective or safe sunscreen is for very young babies. Keep your baby shaded from the sun by using a parasol

---

or sun canopy on their buggy or pram; keep checking it is still providing shade as the sun moves around during the day, and adjust it if necessary. If you have to carry your baby when out and about in the sun, a sun hat will protect their face, neck and ears. Make sure their skin, including their arms and legs, is covered with lightweight cotton clothing. Remember your baby can quickly become dehydrated in hot weather so offer them breast milk, or if they are formula fed, cooled boiled water, frequently.

Going on holiday with your baby

If you want to take your baby on holiday in the first three months there are a few points to consider. If you are planning on going abroad, most airlines are happy for babies to fly from two days old, perhaps with a letter from your GP stating your baby is fit to fly; some will only allow babies to fly from the age of two weeks onwards. If your baby was born prematurely, you must count their age from their due date, not from the date they were born. Also, if you had a Caesarean section you aren't allowed to fly for the first ten days.

One of the great advantages of going on holiday while your baby is very young rather than when they become mobile is that they are much easier to transport and there are far fewer safety concerns, but it's probably best to wait a few weeks before flying, to give you and your partner time to get to know your new arrival. Also, your baby's immune system is immature during the first few weeks, so you might not want to expose them to other travellers' germs at that time.

Avoid taking your baby to countries where there are diseases they are too young to be vaccinated against. For example, if your baby is under two months old it's not safe for them to take anti-malarial medicine. Always check with your GP first if you're planning to take your baby to a destination where vaccinations are needed.

If your baby has a cold or an ear infection their ears are more likely to feel uncomfortable during the flight due to the changing air pressure when taking off and landing. If you have any concerns, check with your GP before flying. A good way of reducing ear discomfort is to breast or bottle-feed your baby during take-off and landing, as the sucking action helps to push air into the middle ear, which helps to even up the pressure, thus preventing or easing any pain.

Many airlines will charge for your baby to fly, even though they will be sitting on your knee secured in a special safety belt during the flight, so you will need to buy them a ticket; though often the fare is greatly reduced, or even free, for babies who will be aged under two on the return journey.

If you are flying abroad babies will need their own passport. Ask if you can pre-book a travel cot for your baby, or if you can take your baby's car seat onboard for them to sit in. Most airlines – even low-cost carriers – will allow you to check in one pushchair and car seat free of charge and sometimes a travel cot as well (although check with the airline carrier before booking your flight); you can usually give the pushchair to airline staff at the boarding gate to be stored in the hold. Many airlines allow you to keep the pushchair with you until you reach the steps of the aircraft. The majority of airlines provide changing tables in the toilets and have bottle-warming facilities on board.

It's also a good idea to check whether your hotel or holiday company can provide any baby equipment, some will provide travel cots and even baby baths and changing mats, which will reduce the amount of equipment you need to take with you.

Breastfeeding on the move

Most UK airports provide chairs in the baby change areas for you to sit on while breastfeeding. Airlines are usually happy for mums to breastfeed their babies during a flight, but it's best to check your airline's policy before booking your holiday. Avoid sitting on an aisle seat so that you can breastfeed discreetly.

It's probably a good idea to pack an extra top in your hand luggage in case of any leaks during or after feeding. If you are uncomfortable about feeding in a public place, another option is to take some expressed milk with you to feed your baby with on the aeroplane.

Stephanie told me: 'Jack was two months old when we flew to Mallorca. I didn't like breastfeeding in front of strangers, so I stored a bottle of breast milk in a cooler bag with ice cubes to keep it cold. I also took a flask of hot water and just warmed the milk when Jack needed it during the flight.'

Bottle-feeding on the move

The easiest way to bottle-feed your baby on the move is with ready-to-use formula, which you can buy in handy little cartons; these are a bit more expensive than powdered baby milk, but they offer a much more convenient way of ensuring your baby has hygienically-prepared milk whenever it's needed during your journey.

If you are flying, the hand luggage restrictions on liquids don't apply to your baby's milk – in most cases you will be able to take up to 1 litre in total of bottles or cartons of prepared milk in your hand luggage – but you should double check with the airline before you fly. However, be aware that airport security may ask you to open a carton, or bottle and taste the contents. Remember to take some sterilised bottles in a sterilised, lidded container as well. If you prefer, you can pre-order cartons of ready-made baby milk from Boots in all UK airports and collect them in the departure lounge, after check-in. You can ask for hot water to warm a bottle in at an airport cafe or restaurant; once on board you can ask a member of the cabin crew to warm a bottle.

You can feed your baby ready-to-feed formula at room temperature, or if you are travelling by car you could use a travel bottle warmer that plugs into your car's cigarette lighter. Alternatively you could take a flask of hot water and a large plastic bowl or jug – you could also do this when travelling by train.

Tip

Note: Never keep made-up formula warm in an insulated carrier, as keeping the milk warm will encourage bacteria growth.

If you prefer, you can make up a feed as and when you need it. To do this you will need to take sterilised bottles, a flask of freshly boiled water and formula powder with you. The water needs to be stored at a temperature of 70°C or above to kill any harmful bacteria. If the flask is filled and kept sealed, the water will stay above 70°C for several hours. You can buy sterile disposable bottles – though these can be quite expensive. Little pots that can hold up to three measures of formula are also available and save the hassle of having to count scoops of milk powder while on the move; always sterilise these before each use.

Always check the temperature of the milk before feeding it to your baby, even if the water has been in a vacuum flask for a few hours. Pour a few drops of milk on to your inner wrist. The milk should feel just warm, not hot. If the bottle is too hot, hold it under a cold tap (if one is available) ensuring the water doesn't touch the teat. Alternatively leave it to cool down and then check the temperature again.

Throw away leftover milk

You shouldn't keep any formula or breast milk leftover from a feed for longer than an hour as bacteria can breed fast and cause tummy upsets. So if your baby doesn't finish their bottle within an hour throw away any remaining milk.

Holiday essential extras checklist

Below is a handy checklist of some essential extras you might want to take on holiday.

☐ **Passport** – your baby will need their own passport to be able to travel. For further information go to the HM Passport Office page at www.gov.uk.

☐ **Parasol** – to keep your baby shaded from the sun. Remember babies under six months of age shouldn't be exposed to the sun.

☐ **Travel cot –** unless you can reserve one at your holiday accommodation before you go.

☐ **Plug-in night-light** – handy for night feeds and nappy changes.

☐ **Baby monitor –** if, for example, you intend to sit out on the balcony while your baby is asleep in your hotel room.

☐ **Travel blackout blinds** – to block out sunlight if your baby has a nap during the day.

☐ **A universal bath plug –** to turn a washbasin or shower into a baby bath.

CHAPTER 4
CALM YOUR CRYING BABY

The only way your newborn baby can communicate with you is by crying. Crying is designed to grab your attention and ensure that you're aware that your baby needs you. In the early days the number one reason your baby will cry is likely to be in response to hunger. Though of course your baby may cry for many other reasons – including being in a wet or soiled nappy, being overtired, or discomfort from colic, nappy rash, or perhaps thrush. In most cases your baby will stop crying as soon as their needs are met. However, sometimes you won't be able to work out why your baby is crying and you'll need to find ways to soothe them. The important thing is not to worry or feel inadequate if your baby cries a lot – some babies do. So long as they are gaining weight and appear healthy and you always respond to their crying, it won't do them any harm.

Some experts call the first three months of a baby's life 'the fourth trimester' because it is thought that babies need similar conditions to those they experienced in the womb, to help them make the transition to the outside world. Your baby sucked their thumb and fingers from about the fifth month of pregnancy and felt snug and secure in their mother's womb. They experienced movement as you went about your daily life. They heard the noises made by the inner workings of your body, such as the thud of your heart beating, the rumbling of your digestive system and the sound of your voice, as well as external noises such as your partner's voice, music, the vacuum cleaner, the washer and road traffic. They were also aware of your smell. So it follows that the most effective ways of soothing your baby involve re-creating the security, movement, sounds and smells they experienced in the womb. Remember, all babies are different – what works for one might not work for another, so this chapter offers you a range of tried-and-tested techniques to help you calm your crying baby.

In this chapter:

- ▶ Crying baby checklist
- ▶ Offer the breast or a dummy
- ▶ Should I give my baby a dummy?
- ▶ Hold your baby close
- ▶ Rock your baby
- ▶ Carry your baby in a sling
- ▶ Try swaddling
- ▶ Swaddling dos and don'ts
- ▶ Cut crying with massage
- ▶ Make a noise!
- ▶ Cope with crying
- ▶ Be alert to changes in your baby's crying
- ▶ A first-time mum's experiences of crying and how she coped

Crying baby checklist

When your baby cries you need to check for obvious reasons first, such as:

Hunger – check if they are hungry by offering them the breast or a bottle.

Wet or soiled nappy – check their nappy to make sure it isn't wet or soiled.

Sore bottom – check their bottom in case they have nappy rash.

Being too hot – if they seem hot, check their temperature and perhaps remove some clothing to help them cool down.

Being in pain or distress – check for signs they may be suffering from wind, colic, an ear infection or dehydration. For more information on all these and more conditions see Chapter 6 – Home Nurse.

If your baby continues to cry for no apparent reason they may simply be overtired and over-stimulated and unable to fall asleep, in which case one of these soothing methods may help to calm them.

Offer the breast or a dummy

Babies find sucking comforting, so offering them your breast or a dummy could help to soothe them; breastfed babies often suck on the breast without getting milk, simply for comfort – this is known as non-nutritive feeding. If you are breastfeeding avoid offering your baby a dummy in the first few weeks, as it could confuse them and cause problems with breastfeeding (see below). The effort of sucking – especially on the breast – is also tiring and encourages sleep. Another option is to encourage your baby to suck their thumb – most children stop once they have learned other ways of comforting themselves – usually by the age of three of four.

Should I give my baby a dummy?

Most babies are content with feeding and cuddling and don't need a dummy, especially if you are breastfeeding on demand. Some babies won't take a dummy at all while others – breastfed or not – seem to need the extra comfort of sucking on one. You might not be a fan of dummies, but many parents find them a godsend when their baby won't stop crying. If you decide to try your baby with a dummy it may be a case of trial and error before you find one that your baby will take.

Most dummies have a silicone or rubber teat and a plastic or silicone handle and mouth shield designed to prevent your baby from swallowing or choking on the teat. Some are constructed so they have no joins or cracks that could come apart or collect germs. Latex or rubber dummies are softer and more pliable than silicone, but they aren't as long lasting.

Orthodontic dummies are flatter than the more old-fashioned, cherry-shaped dummies. They are designed to encourage the same type of sucking action that babies use when they breastfeed and to be less likely to affect the way their teeth develop.

Buy a few dummies so you can change and sterilise them often. You can buy dummies that come with a holder for you to store them in and keep them clean when not in use. For safety and hygiene reasons check your baby's dummies regularly and throw them away if you notice any signs of wear and tear.

To minimise the effects of dummies on how your baby's teeth grow only use them when necessary and try to wean them off them at six months if you can. Never dip your baby's dummy in something sweet like honey or jam, as this could cause tooth decay and some experts think it could encourage a 'sweet tooth'.

Hold your baby close

Holding your baby close to you, whether it is while breast or bottle-feeding, or simply when cuddling them, helps them to feel more secure and relaxed. Snuggled up close your baby can hear the sound of your heartbeat; skin-to-skin contact is especially calming because your baby can inhale your familiar scent. These are all reminders of their time in their mother's womb. When you cuddle your baby they will release the calming hormone oxytocin, which helps to reduce their stress hormone levels; your body also produces oxytocin, so it has a calming effect on you as well, helping to relieve the stress of hearing your baby cry.

Rock your baby

Most babies find movement soothing – again because it re-creates the conditions they encountered in the womb. Rocking your baby gently in your arms or walking around with them cradled in your arms, or held upright with their head resting on your shoulder offers them the calming effects of movement as well as of being held. You can gently rock your baby in their crib, or if you need your hands free you could put them in their bouncing chair and rock them gently using a hand or foot. Pushing your baby backwards and forwards, or gently jiggling them from side to side in their pram or buggy often has the same soothing effect. Some babies settle when taken out for a short car or buggy ride.

Carry your baby in a sling

Carrying your baby in a sling is another way to hold your baby close and calm them through movement. It is useful if you have things to do, because you can settle your baby at the same time, or you could pop out for a walk while carrying them in a sling.

Try swaddling

Swaddling is a centuries-old technique that involves wrapping a baby in a cover to help them feel safe and secure as they did in the womb. It's especially good for calming your baby when they are tired but unable to sleep because they are over-stimulated, but bear in mind some babies don't seem to like being swaddled.

How to swaddle your baby

Below is a step-by-step guide to swaddling your baby.

1. Spread a cot sheet on the floor in a diamond shape.

2. Fold the top corner over about 15 cm deep to make a flat edge.

3. Lie your baby on their back on the sheet, with their neck resting on the flat edge.

4. Pull the left corner over your baby's body and tuck it under their bottom.

5. Bring the bottom corner up to cover your baby's feet.

6. Wrap the right corner across their body and around their back, so that only their head and neck are left uncovered.

Swaddling dos and don'ts

Do leave enough room for your baby to draw their legs up into the 'frog' position with their thighs held roughly at right angles to their body, as this allows the hips to develop correctly. If their legs are swaddled too tightly in a 'straight down' position it may cause or worsen a condition known as hip dysplasia, where the hips don't work properly because they aren't properly aligned.

Don't use a blanket to swaddle your baby, as this could lead to them overheating, which is a risk factor for sudden infant death syndrome (SIDS).

Don't swaddle your baby while breastfeeding, as they are more likely to overheat. Also, research suggests that babies use their hands to find the breast and latch on, so swaddling during breastfeeds could lead to feeding problems.

Don't lie your baby down on their front when swaddled.

Don't swaddle your baby once they start waving their arms and kicking their legs, as it may hamper their mobility and development.

Cut crying with massage

Baby massage has been practised all over the world for centuries and has been shown to reduce crying and improve sleep quality. We instinctively touch our babies when they cry – for example to cuddle them or rub their back. Massage is simply a progression of this inbuilt impulse. The skin-to-skin contact helps your baby to feel safe and secure and it stimulates the release of calming oxytocin in you and your baby, lowering stress levels and promoting calm. It also encourages the production of relaxing serotonin and pain-relieving endorphins, so it can help to ease wind and colic. If your baby is constipated a gentle tummy massage can help provide relief. Massage also offers a hands-on opportunity for you or your partner to bond and interact with your baby. It's a good way for dads to spend some quality time with their babies – maybe as part of your baby's bedtime routine, as it can help you both relax at the end of the day. If you or your partner suffers from postnatal illness (PNI), massaging your baby can help to relieve your symptoms and improve your relationship with your baby.

Baby massage has been linked to other benefits, such as boosting your baby's circulation, promoting weight gain and encouraging mental and emotional development.

Oils and creams suitable for baby massage

An oil or cream makes it easier to glide your hands over your baby's skin and helps to moisturise and protect their skin.

You could use baby oil, or baby massage oil – many of which contain relaxing essential oils like lavender or chamomile. Sunflower, coconut, grapeseed or sweet almond oils are also fine. Avoid using olive oil for massage as it contains oleic acid, which can damage your baby's delicate skin barrier. Aqueous cream isn't recommended either as it contains sodium lauryl sulphate, a harsh detergent that could also irritate your baby's skin. If your baby has eczema it might be advisable to use the emollient cream your GP has prescribed.

Simple baby massage

Below are some simple baby massage guidelines. You should perform each technique up to three times on each side.

1. Choose a time when your baby is content and alert, not hungry or tired, for example just before the bedtime feed.

2. Gather together everything you'll need – a changing mat with a towel on top, your chosen massage oil or cream, a change of baby clothing and your usual nappy-changing kit.

3. Loosen or remove your baby's nappy and clean their bottom if necessary.

4. Warm some of your chosen oil or cream in your hands.

5. Gently hold one of your baby's ankles with one hand and glide your other hand up the front of their leg and then down the back. Repeat on the other leg.

6. Hold one foot and use your thumbs to massage the sole in little circles. Gently squeeze each toe. Repeat on the other foot.

7. Place both hands lightly on your baby's tummy. With your hands relaxed gently stroke their tummy in big clockwise circles.

8. Gently glide both hands in an outward circular motion from the middle of their chest across the shoulders, and then back around to the chest. Gently slide your hands down each arm.

Safe massage

Avoid massaging your baby if they are unwell, have a temperature, or have just had vaccinations. Stop massaging if your baby seems upset, or falls asleep.

Make a noise!

It might sound counterproductive, but making a noise might help to settle your baby. Everyday noises your baby heard when they were in the womb, such as the sound of the television, radio, vacuum cleaner, washing machine, dishwasher or tumble dryer can help to soothe and calm them. You could try vacuuming while carrying your baby in a sling, or put them in a bouncing chair where they can watch you. You could turn on the radio, to see if the music settles them. The familiar sound of your voice can be calming, so try talking or singing to your baby when they are upset.

Cope with crying

You may have days where your baby cries more than usual – perhaps because they are suffering with colic, for example – and you feel like you've had enough. If this happens, try these strategies to help you cope:

1. Breathe in deeply to a count of five, hold your breath to a count of five, and then exhale to a count of five.

2. If you are alone, place your baby safely in their Moses basket, pram or cot, then take a break by going into another room and sitting down. You might want to make yourself a hot drink and watch TV or listen to the radio – anything that will help you relax and calm down for 5 minutes or so before returning to your baby.

3. Ask your partner or a family member if they could look after your baby for a while; even just an hour or so away from your baby could be enough to recharge your batteries and help you cope.

4. Babies usually cry less by the time they reach three months, so remind yourself, 'this too shall pass'.

5. If none of these strategies help and your baby's crying is getting you down, seek help; talk to your health visitor about how you are feeling, or ring a helpline such as Cry-sis, Family Life, or Home Start. For further details of these organisations see the Directory, page 198.

Be alert to changes in your baby's crying

If your baby changes the way they cry, it could be a sign that they are poorly. If they suddenly start crying more often than usual and can't be comforted, or if their cry becomes weaker, or more high-pitched, seek medical advice immediately.

A first-time mum's experiences of crying and how she coped

Stephanie, 30 – first-time mum to Sophie

'At first Sophie seemed to cry for three reasons – when she was tired, when she was hungry and when she needed her nappy changing. I usually knew which one it was. Once Sophie was about six weeks old she would sometimes cry for a cuddle. Sometimes she got overtired and needed help to get to sleep. After a few weeks I got used to it.

'I introduced a dummy when Sophie was about two weeks. I was reluctant at first – I'd had it drilled in my head that dummies were bad, but it was the best thing I ever did. Once I found a dummy she was happy with, it settled her straight away.

'I was told in hospital to change my baby's nappy before feeding her, in order to wake her up, so I always changed her first, then fed her and then she usually went back to sleep – so the three main things were ticked off. Once she was about eight weeks old, I would change her, feed her, play with her, then get her to sleep. Sometimes play would go on for too long and she would get overtired, but because I had a little routine I could guess why she was crying and help her get to sleep; if all else failed a cuddle would usually settle her. So my advice would be to try to get a little routine and go through your mental checklist.'

CHAPTER 5
SWEET DREAMS

Sleep – yours, your partner's and your baby's, is another issue that is likely to dominate your first few months of parenthood. Understanding how to help your baby to develop good sleeping habits, so that you and your partner can have a reasonable amount of sleep, is important for everyone's well-being. In the first three months you can expect to suffer from disrupted sleep due to night-time feeds, but there are ways of minimising the impact, so that you are able to cope until your baby starts sleeping for longer stretches during the night.

In this chapter:

- ▶ Your baby's sleep – what to expect
- ▶ How to encourage good sleep habits
- ▶ Settling your baby to sleep
- ▶ Deciding whether or not to co-sleep
- ▶ Co-sleeping dos and don'ts
- ▶ Dealing with sleep-deprivation
- ▶ First time parents' experiences of sleep-deprivation
- ▶ Don't try to be a domestic goddess

Your baby's sleep – what to expect

Newborn babies usually sleep quite a lot, around 16 hours on average, but they don't tend to follow a particular pattern. They will wake often during the day and night because their stomachs are so small they need frequent feeds – especially if you are breastfeeding. Babies also have a shorter sleep cycle than adults, so they have lighter, more easily disturbed sleep. Also, they haven't yet developed a sleep/wake cycle that is influenced by things like daylight and darkness, diet and exercise, so you can expect to be woken up quite often during the night.

At six to eight weeks your baby will tend to sleep for shorter periods during the day and longer spells at night. However they will still wake up for feeds during the night. They will begin to develop a longer sleep cycle with more deep, non-REM sleep and less light sleep[15].

While some babies start sleeping through the night at eight weeks, it's likely that your nights will continue to be disturbed until they are a few months old. But even at this early stage, you can start encouraging good sleeping habits, which will eventually lead to an established sleep routine.

How to encourage good sleep habits

Babies need their sleep just like adults. Below are some steps you can take to help ensure they get sufficient sleep and start to associate night-time with sleep and daytime with wakefulness.

Recognise when your baby is tired

For the first few weeks your baby probably won't stay awake for more than a couple of hours at a time. Recognising when they are tired and encouraging them to sleep will avoid them becoming overtired and fretful. Your baby may yawn, have drooping eyelids, or they may rub their eyes, pull their ears or hair, or start fussing or crying and looking for the comfort of a feed, when they are feeling sleepy. You'll soon know instinctively when they are ready for sleep.

Teach your baby the difference between night and day

Once your baby is around two weeks old you can start teaching them the difference between night and day.

During the day

Change your baby's clothes each morning when they wake up, so they link getting dressed with daytime. Play with them so they associate activity with daytime. Talk to them to encourage them to stay awake and alert. Take them outdoors in the daylight to encourage their body to stop producing the sleep hormone melatonin and to release it at night.

Encourage your baby to sleep through daytime noise.

Your baby was used to hearing noises when they were in the womb, and quite often familiar sounds such as the washing machine, vacuum cleaner, dishwasher or TV will help them to settle down and go to sleep, so don't feel you have to be quiet during their daytime naps. If you creep around you will probably find that as they get older they wake up at the slightest noise, making life difficult for you and your partner.

At bedtime

Develop a regular night-time routine such as a bath, followed by a massage, a bedtime story or song, then a breastfeed or bottle and bed. This will give your baby time to wind down before bed. Your baby's brain will gradually become programmed to associate these events with sleep. Also the warm bath will relax them and raise their temperature slightly. The brain tries to reduce the body temperature to slow down the metabolism and conserve energy, so as your baby's temperature falls slightly their brain will get the 'message' that it is time to sleep. Turn the lights down low, so that your baby learns to associate darkness with sleep. It will also encourage their brain to produce the sleep hormone melatonin.

During the night

The key here is to teach your baby that they should be asleep, not wide-awake, during the night, so don't do anything that will stimulate them. Avoid putting the light on during night feeds, if you need some lighting use a lamp with a low wattage bulb to avoid encouraging your baby to wake up. Don't talk to your baby during feeds, even if they seem wide-awake and want to play! Only change their nappy if it is soiled, or very wet.

Encourage your baby to fall asleep independently

Babies often fall asleep while having a breastfeed or a bottle, or while being held and rocked, but problems can arise if they always expect to fall asleep in your arms only to wake up as soon as you put them down in their Moses basket or cot. To avoid this, try to put them down to sleep in their cot while they are still awake, so that they get used to falling asleep themselves. They may cry for a short time and then settle. However, if they don't self-settle after a few minutes and sound upset then pick them up again. Not everyone is comfortable with leaving their baby to self-soothe, and how you feel about it will probably depend on how quickly your baby settles, so you need to decide what suits you both best. However, be warned, if your baby always needs to be fed, cuddled or rocked to sleep, they won't know how to settle themselves back to sleep when they wake up naturally during the night. That means your broken nights may continue for a lot longer than they need to.

Safe sleeping

Always put your baby down on their back to sleep in the 'feet to foot' position – with their feet at the end of their Moses basket, crib or cot. Research shows this is the safest sleeping position, as there is less risk of SIDS.

Deciding whether or not to co-sleep

Bringing your baby into bed with you, also known as co-sleeping, is a contentious issue. Some experts argue that co-sleeping is natural, encourages bonding and means that mums who breastfeed can do so while dozing or even sleeping, which gives them more much-needed rest and helps to promote successful breastfeeding.

However, the children's charity Unicef advises against the practice because it is linked to a higher incidence of SIDS. They argue that research shows that a cot, crib or Moses basket at the side of your bed is the safest place for your baby to sleep at night. They also warn that it is not safe to bed-share in the first few months, if your baby was born very small or pre-term, or is ill or has a fever.

It is for you and your partner to decide whether or not to bring your baby into bed with you. If you do decide to sleep with your baby, in spite of the warnings from Unicef, pay special attention to the dos and don'ts with regard to the practice.

Co-sleeping dos and don'ts

- ▶ **Do** keep your baby away from pillows.

- ▶ **Do** ensure your baby can't fall out of bed, or get stuck between the mattress and wall

- ▶ **Do** use sheets and a lightweight blanket rather than a duvet, to reduce the risk of your baby overheating.

- ▶ **Do** ensure the bedding is well away from your baby's face or head.

- ▶ **Do** lie your baby down on their back, as you would if they slept in a cot, crib or Moses basket.

- ▶ **Don't** leave your baby alone in bed, as they might slip down under the bedding.

- ▶ **Don't** bed-share if you or your partner has consumed alcohol or drugs, or are overtired, as this increases the risk of you inadvertently rolling over onto your baby.

- ▶ **Don't** co-sleep if either or both of you smoke.

▶ **Don't** co-sleep on the sofa or an armchair, as there is a greater risk of your baby becoming trapped between you and the furniture.

Dealing with sleep-deprivation

Doing the night feeds is bound to leave you feeling tired and sleep-deprived. Below are some ways you could grab some extra sleep or at least improve the quality of the sleep you do get.

1. **Ask your partner to take over the night feeds one or two nights a week** when they are not at work the next day – probably at the weekend – then at least you can have one or two nights of uninterrupted sleep. Or ask if they would take over the early morning feed once or twice a week so that you can have a much-needed lie-in. As well as giving you a break, giving your partner a 'turn' to feed your baby will give them a chance to form a closer bond with them. If your baby is being breastfed, you could use expressed milk to give to your baby from a bottle. Kirsty, 29, told me: 'I dreaded going to bed during the week knowing I would have a sleepless night. At the weekend my husband would stay up until 2 a.m. and give Ethan expressed milk from a bottle, so I could get some uninterrupted sleep.'

2. **Sleep when your baby sleeps** at least once during the day.

3. **Go to bed shortly after your baby's last feed of the day.** Even though it's tempting to stay up late to reclaim some 'me

time', it's better to wind down for just an hour or less before making your way to bed. That way, with luck, you should get a 2 or 3-hour stretch of sleep before your baby wakes for their next feed.

4. Practise good sleep habits to help improve your sleep quality. Get up and go to bed at roughly the same time each day and go outdoors during the day to regulate your body clock and help you drop off quicker. Avoid drinking caffeinated drinks such as tea, coffee or cola after 6 p.m. Wind down for a little while before you go to bed – perhaps by watching a programme on TV that helps you switch off, or reading a book. Darkness and a cool temperature encourage sleep, so hang heavy dark curtains or blackout blinds and keep your bedroom at around 16°C. Avoid eating a heavy meal just before bed, as digesting it can keep you awake. Instead have a sleep-inducing snack, such as a glass of milk and a banana, which supply relaxing magnesium, calcium and tryptophan, which your body uses to make the sleep hormone melatonin.

5. Remind yourself your baby will eventually sleep through the night and by three months many babies, whether breast or bottle-fed, will sleep for 5 to 6 hour stretches each night.

First-time parents' experiences of sleep-deprivation

Annie, 30 – first-time mum to Dylan

'Everyone told me to sleep when your baby does. I didn't and I've yet to meet a mother who does. I wish I had, but I tried to do all the things I couldn't do when my baby was awake, like housework, having a bath, having a meal, or a cup of tea.'

James, 30 – first-time dad to Evie

'I work shifts, so the sleep loss wasn't so much of a problem for me, but there were nights when I would get no sleep before work. Those days were the hardest. Coffee helped and having an early night when possible. I'd advise new parents to accept the fact they are going to be sleep deprived at first. Once you do that, things seem easier.'

Don't try to be a domestic goddess

If you're used to holding down a job and running the home you might be tempted to fit in as many household chores as you can while your baby is asleep. However, if you're tired from having your sleep disrupted and your body is still recovering from the birth, now is not the time to try to be a domestic goddess – there'll be plenty of time for that when your baby is older. It is especially important to rest as much as you can when you first go home with your new baby. Below are some tips to help you maintain your home to a reasonable standard in the first few weeks of parenthood.

- Accept all offers of help and don't be frightened to ask for help.

- Lower your standards a little – no one is going to expect your house to be immaculate at all times.

- Rather than trying to tidy up all day, keep a basket in your main living area where you can place items until you have time to put them away later.

- Keep all of your baby's items – e.g. changing mat, nappies, Moses basket – together in one corner of the living room; it will look a lot tidier than having them spread all over.

- Carry your baby around in a sling while you complete a few lightweight chores, like dusting or putting clothes away. If you don't have time to vacuum, just pick up any noticeable fluff, etc.

- 'White noise' e.g. the sound of a vacuum cleaner or hairdryer often sends babies to sleep. So if your baby won't drop off, try doing some vacuuming and tackle two tasks at the same time!

- Don't try to clean the whole house in one go – break it down into manageable chunks, focussing on one room each day.

- On days when you have little time to do anything, target the most important tasks – for example washing the dishes or loading the dishwasher, cleaning the kitchen worktops and the toilet or doing a load of washing. The rest can wait until later.

CHAPTER 6
HOME NURSE

It's likely that your baby will suffer from one minor ailment or another in the first three months. It's hard not to worry when your baby seems unwell, but having some knowledge of the conditions that commonly affect newborns and what you can treat at home and how, as well as being able to recognise when to call the doctor, will help you cope. Being aware of what to do in an emergency is essential for every parent, so this chapter also includes emergency first aid for babies.

In this chapter:

- ▶ Baby acne
- ▶ Breathing problems
- ▶ Colic
- ▶ Conjunctivitis and blocked tear ducts
- ▶ Constipation
- ▶ Coughs and colds
- ▶ Cradle cap
- ▶ Dehydration
- ▶ Diarrhoea
- ▶ Ear infections
- ▶ Eczema
- ▶ Fever
- ▶ Heat rash

- ▶ Nappy rash
- ▶ Thrush
- ▶ Vomiting
- ▶ Immunisation
- ▶ Emergency first aid for babies

Baby acne

If your baby has pimples or blisters and reddish patches of skin on their cheeks, forehead, chin or back, they could have baby acne. Baby acne is fairly common and usually appears within the first couple of weeks after birth. It's thought to be due to your hormones crossing the placenta and causing your baby's sebaceous (oil) glands to clog, similar to the way hormones trigger teenage acne. Baby boys are more likely to develop baby acne than girls. Baby acne usually goes away on its own without any treatment, but it can take a few weeks. If the affected areas seem especially oily then gently clean them with lukewarm water and cotton wool several times a day.

Watch out for other symptoms

Baby acne is harmless and doesn't make your baby ill. So if your baby has spots and develops a temperature above 38˚C or seems unwell, the spots may be a rash rather than baby acne and you should seek medical advice immediately.

Breathing problems

As a new parent you will probably find yourself checking your baby's breathing often when they are asleep. It is normal for your baby to breathe in cycles, with their breaths becoming faster and deeper, then slower and shallower. It is also normal for them to stop breathing for 5 seconds or so, then start again with deeper breaths. Occasional grunting and snorting noises are also normal.

However, if you have any concerns here's how you can check your baby's breathing:

1. **Listen** with your ear next to your baby's mouth and nose for the sound of breathing.

2. **Watch** for your baby's chest going up and down as they breathe in and out.

3. **Feel** by gently placing a finger next to your baby's mouth and nose to check whether air is being expelled.

For extra reassurance you could buy a baby monitor that allows you to listen in on your baby when you aren't in the same room and alerts you if they stop breathing. See Useful Products, page 194.

When to seek medical attention

You should seek immediate medical attention, if your baby:

Has more than 60 breaths a minute.

Grunts after each breath.

Has flared nostrils, which suggests they are making an extra effort to breathe.

Makes a high-pitched rasping sound and has a barking cough.

Stops breathing for longer than 10 seconds.

Has retractions; this is where the rise and fall of their chest is much more pronounced than normal.

Goes blue across their forehead, nose and lips, which suggests a lack of oxygen.

For details of what to do if your baby stops breathing see page 160.

Colic

If your baby cries for long periods and won't be soothed by feeding, rocking or swaddling – especially in the evenings – they may have colic. Colic is simply a term used to describe excessive crying in a baby. Babies with colic also tend to draw their legs up towards their tummy, clench their fists and become red faced. Both breast- and bottle-fed babies can suffer from the condition, which is thought to affect as many as one in four babies.

There are several theories as to the cause or causes of colic, including indigestion, trapped wind, or a temporary sensitivity to certain proteins and sugars found in breast milk and formula milk. Another possible cause of colic is a bacterial imbalance in the gut – especially if there is an excess of 'bad' bacteria such as *E. coli*, which can contribute to colic symptoms by causing wind and bloating. Below are some techniques and treatments that may help to prevent/relieve colic.

Reduce the amount of air your baby takes in during feeds

Hold your baby in a fairly upright position during breast- or bottle feeds.

If you are bottle-feeding check the teat flow isn't too fast for your baby, or use an anti-colic bottle and teat. For more information on bottle-feeding see page 22.

Burp your baby

Sitting your baby upright on your lap and gently rubbing their back in the middle and at the end of each feed (breast and bottle) can help to release any trapped air from their tummy. For more information on feeding your baby see Chapter 2 – Feed Your Baby.

Try over-the-counter remedies

There are several remedies for colic that you can buy over-the-counter. They work by breaking down trapped wind so that your baby can expel it more easily.

Gripe water is an old-fashioned remedy that contains bicarbonate of soda and dill seed oil – however it can only be given to babies from one month old. Other treatments include Infacol Colic Relief Drops, which contains an anti-flatulent called simethicone and is suitable from birth. If these remedies don't help, your baby's colic may be due to a dietary cause – either mum's diet if you are breastfeeding, or your baby's formula milk if you are bottle-feeding.

THE NEW PARENTS' SURVIVAL GUIDE

If you are breastfeeding, check your diet

Sometimes what you eat can trigger colic in your baby. Some babies develop a short-term intolerance to cow's milk protein in your breast milk. Other common culprits include caffeine, broccoli, cauliflower, cabbage, onions and spicy foods. If you suspect something you are eating or drinking is causing the problem, try cutting it out for a week to see if your baby's symptoms improve, but speak to your GP first if you think it may be caused by dairy foods. If you decide to go dairy-free you will need to make sure you eat other sources of calcium such as almonds, Brazil nuts, tinned sardines (including the bones), dried apricots, dates and figs.

If you are bottle-feeding, try a hypoallergenic milk formula

If you are bottle-feeding and are worried that your baby has an intolerance to cow's milk protein, ask your health visitor or GP about changing to a hypoallergenic (hydrolysed) milk formula in which the proteins have been broken down so they are less likely to cause problems. For more information about formula milks see page 72.

Try probiotics

Probiotics have been shown to help reduce colic. They seem to work best for breastfed babies, but they are still worth trying if you are bottle-feeding. The type of probiotic used in recent research was *Lactobacillus reuteri* and is available in the UK in drop form. For more information see Useful Products, page 194.

When to seek medical advice

If none of these suggestions help it's worth seeing your doctor – just in case there's an underlying problem, such as a hernia. If your doctor is satisfied there is no underlying cause they may prescribe an anti-spasmodic. If nothing helps, try not to worry – colic usually settles down by the age of three to four months.

If your baby suffers from diarrhoea, vomiting or a raised temperature (over 38°C), or if you are not sure if your baby is suffering from colic, see your health visitor, midwife or doctor as soon as possible.

Conjunctivitis and blocked tear ducts

If you notice your baby's eye is pink and watery, or has a yellow discharge they may have conjunctivitis. Conjunctivitis can be caused by an allergy or by a viral infection. If your baby is under one month old take them to see your GP straight away as in very young babies conjunctivitis could be due to a more serious infection.

Another cause of conjunctivitis is a blocked tear duct. Blocked tear ducts are quite common in new babies and are usually due to the duct not being fully developed. This means tears from their eyes can't drain away, which can make their eyes watery and sticky.

Remove any discharge by bathing your baby's eyes using cotton wool dipped in breast milk or cooled boiled water; the breast milk works because it contains antibodies and probiotics. If your baby's conjunctivitis is caused by an infection dispose of the cotton wool immediately and wash your hands, as infective conjunctivitis is highly contagious.

Encourage the blocked tear duct to open up by gently massaging both sides of your baby's nose, working from the top down. This can help to disperse the tears in the blocked duct and may also help the tear duct to develop. In most cases the tear duct will open up after a few weeks and the watering and stickiness will stop, though occasionally it can take months.

Constipation

If your baby passes small, hard, pellet-like poos and is straining to pass them they may be constipated. Your baby may also appear in pain and cry before having a poo. They may have offensive-smelling wind and poo and their tummy may feel solid. Having fewer than three poos in a week is another sign your baby may be constipated. However, in breastfed babies infrequent poos can be perfectly normal. They are generally less likely to suffer from constipation than babies who are formula-fed because breast milk is much easier to digest.

Also, strangely, runny poo can sometimes be a symptom, as it can slip past the hard poo that is causing the blockage.

Watch out for other symptoms

If your baby is not producing many wet nappies, or their fontanelles or eyes appear sunken, their constipation may be due to dehydration (see 'Dehydration' on page 142). If they seem to be in a lot of pain, have a fever, or are passing bloody stools, see a doctor immediately as the constipation could be a sign of food poisoning, a metabolic disorder, a congenital or other condition.

The following steps may help to relieve your baby's constipation.

▶ If your baby is breastfed offer them more feeds.

▶ If your baby is formula-fed give them extra drinks of cooled boiled water. Also check that you are preparing their bottles correctly, as using too much milk powder could cause constipation.

▶ Help to get things moving by gently massaging your baby's tummy in a clockwise direction, with a little baby oil or lotion. If your baby seems distressed, stop immediately.

▶ Gently rotate your baby's legs in a cycling movement, to encourage the poo to pass through their system.

If none of these home remedies work, see your doctor.

Coughs and colds

If your baby has a cough and a blocked or runny nose along with a raised temperature, they are likely to be suffering from a cold.

Various viruses cause colds and your baby may catch several in their first year because their immune system isn't functioning properly yet.

Reduce the risk of your baby catching a cold

Breastfeeding your baby helps them to ward off infections because it passes on the antibodies your body has produced in response to illnesses. You can also protect your baby by keeping them away from anyone who has a cough or a cold. If that isn't possible, make sure everyone washes their hands before handling your baby. You should also avoid exposing your baby to cigarette smoke, as this makes them more likely to catch colds and take longer to recover from them[16].

Treat your baby's cold

Your baby's cold should go away on its own within a few days. In the meantime, there are a few things you can do to make them feel more comfortable.

▶ Offer your baby extra breast or formula feeds to keep them well hydrated

▶ Clear your baby's blocked or stuffy nose by exposing them to a steamy atmosphere, or using a saline spray or drops, or using a vaporiser. Another option is to remove the mucus using a nasal aspirator.

▶ Apply a small amount of petroleum jelly around the nostrils to soothe any soreness.

When to seek medical attention

You should seek medical advice immediately if your baby:

Has a cold that hasn't improved within three days.

Develops a temperature above 38 ˚C.

Has difficulty breathing.

Has a persistent cough.

Coughs up green, yellow or brown mucus, or it runs from their nose.

Cradle cap

Cradle cap, also known as seborrhoeic eczema, often appears in the first couple of months. It usually appears on the scalp first as thick greasy patches with yellow scales. It can also develop in the armpits, the nose and the nappy area. Although cradle cap looks unpleasant, it isn't itchy or sore and doesn't cause any discomfort, nor is it a sign that your baby will suffer from eczema later on. It usually clears up by itself eventually, but you may find almond oil helps to soften and loosen the scales, so that you can then remove them. Apply a little to the affected areas and leave it to soak in for a few minutes. Then gently remove the scales using a soft baby toothbrush.

Never try to remove the scales with your fingernails, as this could cause an infection. If the affected areas start to weep, bleed, or fill with pus, see your doctor immediately, as the skin may have become infected.

Dehydration

Dehydration is fairly common in babies because their small size makes them more sensitive to fluid loss. There are various causes of dehydration in babies. Fever is one of the most common causes because sweating leads to fluid loss, and faster breathing so your baby exhales more moisture. Overheating due to hot weather, wearing too many layers of clothing or covers, or being in an overly warm room could also lead to fluid loss through sweating.

Diarrhoea and vomiting can also cause dehydration[17]. Diarrhoea prevents your baby absorbing fluids in their bowel. Vomiting stops them from keeping fluids in their body.

If your baby is ill they might refuse to have a feed, which can quickly lead to dehydration.

Top tips to prevent dehydration

Don't allow your baby to overheat – see also page 98.

In hot weather offer your baby more frequent breastfeeds, or extra water if they are bottle-fed.

If your baby is refusing feeds because they have an ear infection, take steps to ease the pain (see also 'Ear infections' on page 146.

If your baby is refusing feeds because they have a stuffy nose use a nasal saline wash to help clear it (see also 'Coughs and colds' on page 139).

Signs that your baby is dehydrated

If your baby is dehydrated they may:

- ► Have dry skin or lips.
- ► Have a sunken fontanelle (the soft spot on the top of your baby's head).
- ► Produce fewer wet nappies than usual.
- ► Have sunken eyes.
- ► Cry without producing tears.
- ► Produce urine that is darker than usual.
- ► Appear lethargic and drowsy.
- ► Breathe more rapidly than usual.
- ► Have cold and blotchy hands and feet.

If you think your baby is dehydrated

Seek medical advice as soon as you can. The doctor will recommend a suitable treatment. In most cases dehydration can be treated at home with an oral rehydration solution, such as Dioralyte, that you can buy over the counter at your local pharmacy or your GP can prescribe. Oral rehydration solutions contain sodium, potassium and glucose, to replace lost fluids, minerals and sugars.

Don't give your baby water alone if they are dehydrated as it can dilute the already low level of minerals in their body and make the problem worse.

Diarrhoea

If your baby passes frequent, watery poos they may have diarrhoea. Bear in mind that the occasional liquid poo is normal and most newborns do poo a lot. Also, breastfed babies tend to produce frequent fairly liquid poos, some after every breastfeed, but they are actually less likely to be a sign of diarrhoea because breast milk boosts 'good bacteria' in their gut, meaning they are less likely to suffer from it than formula-fed babies.

Spotting the signs

It is likely your baby has diarrhoea if:

▶ Their poo is runnier than usual.

▶ Their poo has a more unpleasant smell than usual.

▶ They are pooing more often than usual.

▶ Their poo spurts from their bottom.

▶ They have other symptoms such as vomiting and a fever, or there is blood or mucus in their poo.

Causes of diarrhoea

The most common cause of diarrhoea is a tummy bug, which in babies is usually caused by a virus called rotavirus. Sometimes the rotavirus can cause a serious bowel infection and dehydration. You will be offered a vaccination against rotavirus for your baby when they are eight weeks old and again when they are 12 weeks.

Your baby could also develop diarrhoea due to food poisoning caused by poor hygiene when making up formula feeds, if they are on antibiotics, or if they have an allergy to milk protein.

How to treat your baby's diarrhoea

Diarrhoea caused by a tummy bug usually settles down on its own within a few days, once the infection has cleared. However, if your baby has diarrhoea (with or without vomiting) they can quickly lose too much fluid and become dehydrated, so it is important to ensure they have plenty of breast feeds or formula feeds and extra drinks of cooled boiled water to prevent this. You could also offer your baby sips of an oral rehydration solution to prevent them becoming dehydrated. If you're bottle-feeding make sure you are sterilising the equipment properly. For more information on sterilising see page 74.

Don't give your baby fruit juices or glucose drinks – these could make their diarrhoea worse.

Don't give your baby an anti-diarrhoeal medicine – these are unsuitable for children under 12 years of age.

See your doctor straight away, if your baby's diarrhoea:

- ▶ Is accompanied by vomiting.
- ▶ Lasts for more than 24 hours.
- ▶ Contains blood or mucus.
- ▶ Has a jelly-like consistency.

Or if:

▶ You think your baby is dehydrated – see also 'Dehydration' on page 142.

▶ You suspect your baby has a milk allergy.

Ear infections

Ear infections often follow a cold. With young babies the main symptoms are pulling away from the breast or bottle during feeds because sucking is painful, fever and crying that you can't calm. They may rub or pull at their ear and, in severe cases, there may be a discharge from the ear.

It your baby is reluctant to feed offer them more frequent but shorter feeds to prevent dehydration. If you think your baby might have an ear infection you should see your GP immediately. A virus causes most ear infections so antibiotics aren't usually helpful. But if your GP suspects a bacterial infection they may prescribe an antibiotic.

Ease the pain

Give your baby infant paracetamol if they are two months or older. If they are three months old you can give them baby ibuprofen or paracetamol. Always follow the dosage instructions on the pack.

Warm a flannel or muslin cloth on a radiator and hold it against the affected ear for a few minutes at a time, several times a day to help to relieve the pain.

Prevent ear infections

If you are breastfeeding eat more garlic; this will pass on to your baby via your milk and may help to boost their immune system.

When you feed your baby hold them in a fairly upright position, to prevent milk travelling into their ear tube and causing infections.

Avoid letting your baby suck on a dummy for long periods as this may send bacteria from the mouth into the Eustachian tubes between their throat and ears.

Avoid exposing your baby to cigarette smoke as it increases the risk of them developing ear infections.

Eczema

Eczema in babies is fairly common – it is thought to affect up to one in five children before the age of two. The symptoms are reddened, dry, itchy patches that can appear on the face, behind the ears, and in the neck, knee and elbow creases. If it is very itchy your baby is likely to scratch it, which can lead to the skin cracking, bleeding and becoming infected.

Eczema can be inherited, and it tends to run in families. Dry skin is also a key factor – babies' skin tends to be drier than adults' because their oil-producing sebaceous glands haven't yet fully developed. This could help explain why most babies grow out of the condition; over two thirds of children are eczema-free by the time they are seven years old and three quarters of children will be free of the condition by the time they reach 16 years.

If you suspect your baby has eczema you should see your health visitor or doctor. However there are several steps you can take to help prevent and treat flare-ups.

Keep your baby's skin well moisturised – preventing dryness is key to preventing eczema flare-ups. Apply an emollient cream such as Oilatum to their skin several times a day.

Tip Use an emollient when you give your baby a massage. For how to give your baby a massage see page 115.

Don't bath your baby every day during a flare-up – this can make the dryness and itching worse. Instead bath your baby every other day and 'top and tail' them in between.

Use plain lukewarm water or a mild fragrance-free baby wash to clean your baby's skin – perfumed products could cause dryness and irritation. You could also add a bath emollient such as Balneum Bath Oil (see Useful Products, page 194) to the water.

Try an oat bath – oats are known to moisturise the skin, calm inflammation and ease itching. Place a handful of oats in a clean muslin cloth or handkerchief and tie tightly. Drop the bundle into your baby's bath and squeeze it to release the beneficial ingredients. If you prefer a less messy option you could use Aveeno bath and shower oil, which contains oatmeal – though this is only recommended from three months. For more information see Useful Products, page 194.

Use non-biological detergents for washing your baby's clothes, towels and bedding – again to avoid irritating their delicate skin.

Dress your baby in cotton clothes – this prevents them from getting too hot, which can exacerbate the itching and also avoids irritating the skin.

Put scratch mittens on your baby – these prevent them from irritating the skin any further; or keep their nails short to limit the effects of scratching.

Use a one per cent steroid cream to soothe a flare up – these can be bought over the counter and are safe to use on babies. Only use them in small amounts and for short periods until the flare-up has settled down, as prolonged or excessive use could thin the skin.

Continue breastfeeding for at least the first six months – according to the National Eczema Society this can reduce the severity of your baby's eczema.

If you breastfeed and suspect a particular food is the culprit – speak to your health visitor or doctor as they may suggest excluding a particular food – e.g. cow's milk for two or three weeks to see if your baby's skin improves. However, if you cut out dairy include non-dairy sources of calcium in your diet, such as almonds, apricots and tinned sardines (including the bones).

Fever

A fever is where the body raises its temperature as a natural defence against a viral or bacterial infection, such as a cold, flu or an ear infection. While fevers are normally nothing to worry about, they are relatively rare in young babies, so in the first three months, if your baby develops a temperature of 38°C or more, see a doctor immediately.

You will probably know if your baby has a high temperature just by touching them. They may also look flushed and feel clammy. But you may want to use a thermometer to confirm your suspicions. A digital thermometer is the easiest and most accurate type to use at home. To take a reading, place it under your baby's armpit, with their arm at their side. Ear thermometers are very accurate, but are much harder to use, and strip thermometers aren't recommended because they only tell you your baby's skin temperature.

Your baby may go off their feeds while they have a fever, but make sure you offer them frequent breast or formula feeds to prevent them from dehydrating. If your baby is formula fed, offer them cooled, boiled water as well. Signs of dehydration include a sunken fontanelle, dry lips, fewer wet nappies, small, hard poos and darker urine (see also 'Dehydration' on page 142). Dress them as lightly as possible and cover them with a sheet, rather than a blanket or quilt, when you put them in their crib or cot.

If your baby seems upset or very uncomfortable you can give them infant paracetamol if they are two months or older. Once they reach three months you can give them baby ibuprofen. Always follow the dosage instructions on the pack.

Tip

Warning: Do not give your baby aspirin because it could lead to them developing a serious metabolic disorder called Reye's Syndrome.

If your baby develops a rash, make sure you get them checked by a doctor immediately. If the rash doesn't fade when you press on it with a glass, your baby needs urgent medical attention.

Febrile convulsions (fits)

Sometimes a baby with a high temperature will have a febrile convulsion, or fit. During a febrile convulsion your baby's body will stiffen and their arms and legs will twitch. They can last for 5 to 15 minutes.

However, while fits can be terrifying to see, they don't usually cause any harm. During a convulsion remove their dummy (if they have one). If they are in a place where they could fall, move them to a safe, soft surface, placing them on their side with their face turned to one side to prevent them swallowing any vomit and keep their airway open. Don't restrain your baby in any way.

Tip

Warning: If your baby starts having a fit call 999 for an ambulance[18], as it could be a sign of something serious, such as meningitis.

Heat rash

Heat rash is fairly common in new babies. It appears as a bright red pimply rash and can quickly develop if your baby is too hot. Babies are prone to suffering from heat rash because their sweat glands aren't fully developed so when they sweat to cool down the glands become blocked and a rash develops.

To treat heat rash, take steps to cool your baby down. Undress them and give them a tepid bath. Once they've cooled down dress them in fewer layers, or lighter fabrics. Smooth on some calamine lotion to calm the rash down and ease any itching.

If your baby has a rash that doesn't go away when you press a glass on it, or within a day or two, or appears to get worse, or if they develop a temperature of 38°C or above seek medical advice immediately.

Nappy rash

Nappy rash is characterised by red inflamed skin and raised up spots around the bottom and genital area. It is due to the ammonia in your baby's urine and the bacteria in their poo irritating the skin. To prevent or treat nappy rash you need to minimise the length of time your baby's bottom comes into contact with wee and poo.

Change your baby's nappy often – especially after they've wet or pooed it.

Clean your baby's bottom thoroughly – use cotton wool and plain lukewarm water or gentle fragrance and alcohol-free baby wipes for each nappy change. Pat dry afterwards.

Apply a thin layer of barrier cream at each nappy change – this helps to protect your baby's skin from the poo and wee by forming a protective barrier on their skin.

Give your baby some nappy-free time every day – allow the air onto their skin, by putting them on a towel in a warm room.

Another, rarer cause is an allergic reaction to something that has touched your baby's skin, such as a nappy, baby wipe or nappy cream. In these cases, avoid using the suspect product and try an alternative. For example try a different brand of nappy, or nappy cream or use damp cotton wool instead of baby wipes.

If the nappy rash doesn't clear up, or develops yellow pustules see your health visitor or doctor, as it could have developed into thrush (see below) or become infected.

Thrush

If your baby suddenly goes off their feeds and you notice white patches on their tongue, roof of the mouth, gums and insides of their cheeks there's a good chance they are suffering from thrush. Thrush is a yeast infection caused by an overgrowth of the fungus *Candida albicans*, which is usually present in the mouth, at much lower levels. The patches look like milk curds, but when you rub them with your finger they come off to reveal red, raw patches underneath.

It tends to affect babies aged between one and two months, though older babies and toddlers can suffer from it as well. This is because young babies' immune systems are still developing, so it is harder for them to ward off infections. There are a few ways that babies can pick up thrush: they can pick it up from mum during the birth or from breastfeeding; antibiotics are another cause – either if your baby is prescribed them, or if you are taking them and pass them on through your breast milk. Antibiotics not only kill off 'bad bacteria' but the 'good' ones as well, which allows the fungus to multiply.

Although thrush isn't a serious condition it can make your baby's mouth sore and prevent them from feeding properly, which can in turn lead to dehydration. It can also travel through your baby's digestive system to their bottom where it can cause a nappy rash that can take a while to heal[19].

Treating thrush

If you think your baby has thrush take them to see a doctor. They may prescribe an anti-fungal medication for the mouth such as a gel called miconazole, or a liquid called nystatin. If the thrush has caused nappy rash as well, they will also prescribe an antifungal nappy cream. Thrush usually clears up after a week or so of treatment if it doesn't then go back to see your doctor again. If your baby develops a fever seek further medical advice, as this could be a sign of a different infection. If your baby's mouth is so sore it's preventing them feeding, you might want to give them an age-appropriate painkiller.

If your baby is being breastfed, mum and baby could pass the infection back and forth to each other, so you will need to be treated with an antifungal medication as well to stop this from happening. If you have thrush on your nipples they are likely to feel sore, itchy and burning and may be cracked or very red and shiny. For more information about breastfeeding problems see page 56.

> ### Soothe thrush naturally
>
> Apply a solution of one teaspoon of white vinegar in one cup of boiled water to your nipples after each feed. Make a baking-soda solution by dissolving one teaspoon of bicarbonate of soda to one cup of cooled boiled water. Gently apply the solution to the sore patches in your baby's mouth using a cotton bud. If your baby has a thrush infection on their bottom, add two tablespoons of baking soda to their bath to help soothe the soreness and itching. These treatments help to ease the symptoms of thrush but they don't get rid of it, so you'll still need to use an anti-fungal treatment as well.

Vomiting

Babies often vomit in the first few weeks as their digestive systems get used to feeds. Below are the main types and causes of vomiting, how to treat them and when you should see your doctor.

Possetting

This is where your baby brings up a small amount of milk when they burp due to wind and is not a cause for concern.

Reflux

Reflux is where your baby brings up milk and stomach acid when their tummy is full. It happens when the valve at the end of their food pipe, which keeps their feeds in their stomach, isn't fully developed. Around half of babies under three months will suffer to some degree.

If your baby has reflux they may bring up just a little feed or have hiccups and as long as they seem well, this is nothing to worry about; it will usually resolve itself as your baby gets older. If their reflux is severe they may bring up feeds frequently, cough due to the acid in their throat and cry. They may also refuse feeds and fail to gain weight. If this happens, see your health visitor or doctor immediately. They may recommend or prescribe a thickener that can be added to expressed breast milk or formula, or less often, an antacid for babies.

How to prevent/relieve reflux

It can be very upsetting to see your baby in distress, but there are a few things you can do ease your baby's discomfort.

- ▶ Feed your baby little and often so their stomach doesn't get too full.

- ▶ Hold them fairly upright during feeds and for at least half an hour after, to help prevent the milk and acid coming up.

- ▶ If you need to be out and about carry your baby around in a sling to keep them upright.

- ▶ Keep them as still as possible for at least half an hour after feeds. If your baby is formula-fed, they may need to stay still for longer because formula takes longer to digest.

- ▶ Avoid dressing your baby in clothes that are tight around their middle, as this can make the reflux worse.

Tip You can buy foam wedges, which you place under the cot/crib/pram mattress to keep your baby in a slightly raised position while they sleep. If you use these make sure you put your baby in the 'feet to foot' position to prevent them from slipping under the bedding.

Cow's milk allergy or intolerance

If your baby has an allergy or intolerance to cow's milk they may be sick after a feed. The symptoms are very similar to reflux and sometimes cow's milk allergy or intolerance can be the underlying cause of reflux.

If you suspect your baby has milk allergy or intolerance see your doctor. If you are breastfeeding they may suggest cutting out dairy foods for a short time, to see what happens. If your baby is formula-fed they may prescribe a hydrolysed formula. For more information about cow's milk allergy and intolerance see page 73.

Tummy bug

If your baby starts vomiting suddenly, they may have a tummy bug, otherwise known as gastroenteritis; the most common cause in babies is the rotavirus (see also 'Causes of diarrhoea' on page 144). They may also develop diarrhoea. If your baby is three months or under and you think they have gastroenteritis see your doctor. If your baby is being sick a lot they could become dehydrated – especially if they have diarrhoea as well. See also 'Dehydration' on page 142.

An illness or infection

If your baby's vomiting is accompanied by a fever, and other symptoms such as loss of appetite, a rash, lethargy, a stuffy nose or a cough, they may have an ear infection, flu, or a more serious infection like meningitis. If your baby's temperature is 38°C or above or your baby has a rash that doesn't disappear when you press on it with a glass tumbler, see your doctor immediately.

Pyloric stenosis

This is a rare condition (affecting up to four in 1,000 babies) that causes severe vomiting. It happens when the outlet from the stomach into the small intestine (pylorus) becomes thickened, so the milk can't pass through. If your baby has pyloric stenosis they will usually feed well – only to bring up their feed shortly afterwards.

Pyloric stenosis usually starts within the first few weeks, but can appear up to four months after birth. At first your baby may just bring up a little milk, but as the condition progresses less and less milk gets through and the vomiting becomes more forceful with large amounts shooting across the room (projectile vomiting).

If your baby has pyloric stenosis they will quickly lose weight and become dehydrated, so if they show signs of projectile vomiting, it's important to seek treatment urgently. The condition is easily treated with minor surgery.

Immunisation

Immunisation plays a vital role in preventing serious illness. Below is a handy checklist of the vaccines your baby will automatically be offered by your GP's surgery in the first three months of their life.

Two months

5-in-1 (DTaP/IPV/Hib) vaccine – to protect against diphtheria, tetanus, whooping cough (pertussis), polio and *Haemophilus influenzae* type b (known as Hib – a bacterial infection that can cause severe pneumonia or meningitis in young children).

Pneumococcal (PCV) vaccine – to protect against pneumococcal infections, such as pneumonia, septicaemia (blood poisoning) and meningitis, caused by *Streptococcus pneumoniae* bacteria.

Rotavirus vaccine – to protect against rotavirus infection, a common cause of sickness and diarrhoea.

Three months

5-in-1 (DTaP/IPV/Hib) vaccine – second dose (see above).

Meningitis C – to protect against infection by meningococcal group C bacteria, which can cause meningitis and septicaemia.

Rotavirus vaccine – second dose (see above).

Emergency first aid for babies

Knowing what to do in an emergency can give you peace of mind as a new parent.

Choking

If your baby coughs and gasps for breath, or turns red then blue in the face they may be choking. If there is someone with you, get them to call 999. If you are on your own, take the following steps straight away. Only call 999 after you have repeated the steps **three** times.

1. Check inside your baby's mouth and remove any obstruction if you can. Avoid pushing the object further down their throat.

2. If you can't remove the obstruction lie your baby face down along your forearm with their head lower than their chest, cradling their chin with your fingers. Using the heel of your hand give them up to five firm slaps in the middle of their back.

3. After each slap check to see if the obstruction has cleared. Look inside your baby's mouth and remove any obvious object.

4. If they are still choking after five slaps, turn them onto their back – while still supporting them on your forearm – and turn them so that their head is held lower than their chest.

5. Using two fingers give them up to five chest thrusts by pushing inwards and upwards in the middle of their chest one finger's width below their nipple line.

6. After each thrust check to see if the obstruction has cleared by checking inside your baby's mouth and removing any object.

7. Continue with the cycle of back slaps and chest thrusts until qualified help arrives.

What to do if you think your baby has stopped breathing

Watch, listen and feel for signs of normal breathing for no more than 10 seconds.

If your baby is unconscious but breathing normally, hold them in your arms on their side with their head supported and lower than their body while checking they are still breathing. Call 999 for an ambulance, or take your baby to the nearest A&E, and keep on monitoring their breathing until you get medical help.

If your baby is not breathing or having difficulty breathing you will need to perform cardiopulmonary resuscitation (CPR) immediately.

How to perform CPR on your baby

If there is someone with you, ask them to dial 999 for an ambulance while you start CPR. If you are alone, perform CPR for one minute before dialling 999 for an ambulance.

Open the airway

1. Lie your baby down on their back on a firm, flat, surface.

2. Kneel down facing your baby's chest.

3. Ensure your baby's head and neck are in line (i.e. their head is not tilted to the side).

4. Use a finger to gently lift their chin.

Give five rescue breaths

1. Seal your mouth over your baby's mouth and nose.

2. Blow five breaths into your baby's mouth and nose, watching for their chest to rise.

3. When their chest rises, stop blowing and let it fall.

4. Repeat these steps five times.

Watch, listen and feel for signs of normal breathing for no more than 10 seconds. If there are no signs of life start chest compressions with rescue breaths.

Give 15 chest compressions
Place your baby on a firm surface. Place two fingers in the middle of their chest, one finger's width below their nipple line. Press both fingertips down sharply one third of the depth of your baby's chest. Press down 15 times, at a rate of 100 compressions per minute. After 15 compressions, give two rescue breaths.

Continue CPR until the paramedics arrive
Give 15 compressions then two rescue breaths until qualified help arrives. If you can't give rescue breaths for whatever reason, just do the chest compressions.

Keep checking
After each set of 15 compressions and two rescue breaths, watch, listen and feel to see if your baby is breathing again.

CHAPTER 7
BABY MILESTONES –
WHAT TO EXPECT IN THE FIRST THREE MONTHS

One of the things that is most likely to worry you, as a new parent, is whether your baby is developing normally. In this chapter we look at the main developmental milestones of your baby's first three months. However, it is important to remember that the milestones outlined are just a guide – all babies are unique and each will progress at their own rate, so try to resist the temptation to compare your baby's progress to that of others. However, if your baby is unable to do certain things at a particular point in time it could be a sign that something is wrong and further investigation by a health professional may be needed, so I've included a list of 'red flags' for each month. Bear in mind too that if your baby reaches a particular milestone early – for example holding their head up, it won't necessarily mean they'll crawl or walk earlier.

In this chapter:

- ▶ What to expect from your baby:
  - At birth
  - At one month old
  - At two months old
  - At three months old
- ▶ When to seek medical advice
- ▶ How to encourage your baby's development

What to expect from your baby at birth

Your newborn baby will be able to:

▶ See objects around 25 cm to 30 cm away most clearly – this is about the distance between your face and theirs during feeds.

▶ Recognise your voice and other sounds such as the TV, music, the vacuum cleaner etc., having heard them when they were in the womb.

What to expect from your baby at one month old

When your baby reaches four weeks they will be starting to:

▶ Stare at your face.

▶ Notice sounds and stop to listen.

▶ Lift their head for a few seconds when placed on their front.

▶ Stretch out their arms, legs and fingers and gradually unfurl their body from the foetal position.

▶ Follow with their eyes a moving object about 20 cm from their face.

▶ Hold their head steady for a few seconds when you hold them upright.

▶ Make happy sounds like cooing and gurgling.

▶ Smile at you properly – rather than in response to wind!

Babies can't perceive colour very well, so black and white patterns attract their attention the most. You can download black and white geometric patterns from the Internet that can stimulate your baby's visual and brain development. Age-appropriate toys and pictures also stimulate brain development.

Red flags

Every baby develops at their own pace, but see your health visitor or doctor if your one-month-old:

Feeds slowly, or doesn't suck very strongly.

Seems unable to focus their eyes.

Doesn't watch objects moving nearby.

Doesn't respond to bright lights.

Appears stiff or floppy.

Doesn't react to loud sounds.

What to expect from your baby at two months old

When your baby is around eight weeks old they will also be starting to:

▶ Lift their head and upper chest for a little while, when placed on their front.

- ► Wave their arms around and kick with their legs.

- ► Listen attentively to your voice.

- ► Smile back at you when you smile at them.

- ► Chuckle or squeal with pleasure.

- ► Grasp your finger when you place it on their palm.

- ► Mimic your facial expressions, such as frowning, or putting your tongue out.

What to expect from your baby at three months old

When your baby is around 12 weeks they will also be starting to:

- ► Hold their head steady for a few seconds when sat supported on your knee.

- ► Reach out for objects dangled in front of them and sometimes touch them.

- ► Hold and shake a rattle.

- ► Suck their fists and stare at their hands.

- ► Sit up when supported by cushions.

- ► Push themselves up on their arms when lying on their tummy.

- ► Try to roll over.

- ► Try to bear their weight on their legs when supported in a standing position.

> **Red flags**
>
> Every baby develops in their own way, but see your GP if your three-month-old:
>
> Is unable to support their head.
>
> Is unable to grasp objects.
>
> Can't track moving objects.
>
> Doesn't smile.
>
> Fails to react to loud sounds.

How to encourage your baby's development

Here are some ways you can interact with your baby to encourage them to develop their communication and motor skills:

► Give them regular tummy time (see page 95) to allow them to develop their muscles and motor skills.

► Talk and sing to them to encourage them to start trying to communicate with you.

► Tell them what you are doing and name objects around them.

► Read simple stories to them.

► Carry them around and show them objects that might catch their interest.

► Smile at your baby, especially once they start smiling back at you.

- ▶ Once your baby becomes more expressive, try pulling faces and see if they try to copy you.

- ▶ When they start cooing or gurgling at you when you talk, encourage them by pausing and giving them a chance to respond.

- ▶ Repeat the sounds they make back to them.

- ▶ Play peek-a-boo.

- ▶ When they start grasping at objects, offer them a rattle to hold.

CHAPTER 8
LOOK AFTER YOURSELF

It may seem a little strange to include a chapter that is all about looking after yourself in a parenting guide, but remember your baby is relying on you and your partner for their care so it is very important that you are both in the best possible physical and mental shape to provide it. Bear in mind too that your body will have just gone through a massive upheaval after the pregnancy and delivery, so you will be dealing with various physical changes, as well as looking after a new little human being.

So while all your energies will naturally be focussed on caring for your new arrival in the first three months of their life, it is also vital that you and your partner practise good self-care, so that you can both deal with the demands being placed upon you. If either of you are feeling under par or depressed, you will find it much harder to cope. For your own well-being and that of your baby, you and your partner need to take good care of yourselves.

In this chapter:

- ▶ The first few days after the birth
- ▶ Your post-pregnancy body – what to expect
- ▶ Be prepared for the baby blues
- ▶ Recognise postnatal illness (PNI)
- ▶ Be aware of the risk factors for PNI
- ▶ What to do if you think you or your partner have PNI

- ► Eat well
- ► Drink plenty of fluids – but curb the caffeine
- ► Watch your alcohol intake
- ► Take regular gentle exercise
- ► Deal with stress
- ► Real-life tips on surviving early parenthood
- ► And finally…

The first few days after the birth

When I had my first baby new mums were expected to stay in hospital for a week after the birth. While most of us wanted to go home after a couple of days, being in a maternity unit offered many advantages. There were experienced midwives and other staff on hand to help you get to grips with feeding and caring for your baby, all of your meals were made for you and you had no domestic chores to worry about. During that week you had nothing else to do but get to know your baby and rest.

Compare that to today, when most new mums go home within a day of the birth – or after two or three days if you had a forceps delivery or a Caesarean section. The practice of encouraging women to take it easy after the birth was in recognition of the huge physical and emotional upheaval new mums experience and the need to have a period of recovery. So in the first week or two after the birth mums need to remind themselves that this should be a time for doing little else but caring for their baby and resting. Parents shouldn't feel they have to put on a performance for other people and shouldn't have visitors unless they want to. Also they should accept all offers of help to give themselves time to settle into parenthood.

Partners also have to adjust to the pressures of being a parent and will want to play a role in the care of their new baby. Mums should encourage them to be 'hands on' and help with the practical aspects of looking after their new arrival, such as changing nappies, or helping with bath time; even if mum breastfeeds her partner can help by taking over as many of the domestic chores as possible to leave her free to rest and establish her milk supply. After a few weeks partners will also be able to feed expressed milk to their baby via a bottle. As well as helping the mum, it will give them the chance to build an emotional bond with their baby.

Your post-pregnancy body – what to expect

For mums, the first few weeks after the birth of your baby your body will be slowly returning to normal. One of the first things you will notice is that you can see your feet again! Don't expect your body to go back to exactly how it was before you became pregnant. There will be some permanent changes – for example your breasts are likely to be a different shape and size – and your hips may be slightly wider. Here are some of the changes you are likely to experience.

Weight loss

Straight after the birth, you will probably be 11 lb to 22 lb (5–10 kg) lighter; this weight loss will include your baby's weight, the placenta and amniotic fluid, etc. However, if you are breastfeeding your breasts will be heavier. Your stomach is still likely to protrude or be like a saggy pouch with a jelly-like feel to it for the first few weeks at least, until the womb gradually contracts to its pre-pregnancy size – a process known as involution. Avoid the temptation to try to get back in shape too quickly – experts say that it can take as long to lose the weight as it did to put it on. Many women find that breastfeeding helps them to get back to their original size quicker, because it encourages the womb to contract and milk production uses up around 500 extra calories a day. However, not every breastfeeding mum loses the baby-weight straight away so try not to be disappointed if you remain heavier than your pre-pregnancy weight for a while. You can help the process along by avoiding eating extra food – just aim for a balanced, healthy diet.

After pains

In the early days after the birth you will feel 'after pains' as your womb contracts and slowly returns to its normal shape and size. If you breastfeed you'll probably experience quite intense after pains each time you feed your baby. This is because each time you breastfeed your body releases the hormone oxytocin, which stimulates the contractions. After pains feel similar to period pains and should settle down by about the fourth day. If the pain is severe it is safe for you to take an over-the-counter painkiller. Try taking the painkiller 20 minutes or so before each feed so that you can nurse your baby in comfort.

All painkillers you take when breastfeeding will pass on to your baby in tiny amounts through your breast milk. The chart below explains which painkillers are safe to take.

Painkillers for breastfeeding mums checklist

Painkiller	Safe to take when breastfeeding?	Contraindications
Paracetamol	Yes	Speak to your GP before taking if your baby was born before 37 weeks, had a low birth weight or has a medical condition.
Ibuprofen	Yes	Speak to your GP before taking if your baby was born before 37 weeks, had a low birth weight or has a medical condition.
Aspirin	No	Not advised because it could lead to your baby developing a serious metabolic disorder called Reye's Syndrome.

Swollen, tender breasts

Your breasts will feel swollen, tender and hard and look much bigger than usual two or three days after giving birth, due to the milk coming in. If you are breastfeeding your baby will empty your engorged breasts, but if you are bottle-feeding it could take about five days before your body stops producing milk. You can ease the pain by applying cold packs – but avoid warm ones, as these could promote milk production.

Frequent trips to the loo

During pregnancy it is normal for your body to retain water – post-delivery you will start to excrete the extra fluid via sweating and urination – so expect to need to go to the loo more often.

Blood loss

For up to six weeks after the birth you will have a bloody discharge known as lochia, as the uterus shrinks back to normal. It will be bright red and like a heavy period for the first ten days or so before becoming lighter and brownish in colour and then finally a pale yellow. The more you rest the lighter it will be, so this is another reason to take it easy in the first few weeks. If you are breastfeeding you may have heavier blood loss during a feed due to your womb contracting more strongly.

A sore perineum

It is quite common to tear, or need to be cut (i.e. have an episiotomy) during childbirth. The tear or cut will be stitched immediately after the birth and you may have some soreness and pain on the perineum afterwards. Even if you weren't cut and didn't tear, the area may still feel tender. It may also sting when you have a wee. To help alleviate the pain fill a jug with warm water and pour the water over your perineum area as you wee. You might also be worried that having a poo will split your stitches, if you have them – don't worry, it won't, but holding a clean maternity pad over your stitches while having a poo might make you feel more comfortable. Drinking plenty of fluids is also helpful because it keeps your poo soft, so you don't need to strain as much. It also dilutes your urine so it is less likely to sting.

A cut or tear usually takes up to four weeks to heal. To promote healing allow fresh air on the stitches by lying on a towel with your underwear off for 10 minutes a couple of times a day. In the meantime you can safely take an over-the-counter painkiller to relieve the pain (see the chart on page 173).

If you prefer a natural treatment, you may find the homeopathic remedy arnica, which is claimed to reduce bruising and swelling, helps. Putting an ice pack or ice cubes wrapped in a towel on the cut may help to ease the pain. Don't put ice straight on to your skin as it could damage it. Warm baths may also help to reduce the pain and adding a few drops of lavender or tea tree oil can help to promote healing. If you find sitting uncomfortable, you could try using an inflatable cushion designed to ease the pressure on the perineum area when you sit down. These are expensive to buy but you can hire them from the NCT. See also Useful Products, page 194, and the Directory, page 198.

Swollen ankles

Your ankles may be puffy and swollen for the first week or so after the birth. This is because your kidneys may not be able to cope with all of the extra fluid at once, so some of it may build up in your tissues until it can be excreted from your body.

If you had a Caesarean: the scar and soreness

Your scar will be 10 cm to 15 cm long, just below your bikini line. In the first few weeks you will probably experience some pain around the incision and it's likely to feel itchy as it heals, but this should improve within about six weeks. Within a year it will look like a line and be just a shade or two darker than the surrounding skin. In the early days make sure you move around as soon as possible to help you recover more quickly and to prevent blood clots forming.

Postpartum infections

Though rare, childbirth leaves you vulnerable to infections. These can develop in the womb, in the cervix, vagina or on the perineum – due to tears or cuts – or in the wound after a Caesarean section. Symptoms can include fever, pain, or tenderness in the infected area, or a foul-smelling discharge – from the vagina if you have a womb infection – or from a wound. Seek medical help immediately if you experience any of these symptoms.

Stretch marks

Stretch marks are another change you may notice in your body. Massaging your tummy with an oil such as Bio-Oil, both during and after pregnancy, can help to prevent and improve stretch marks – though they usually fade in time from purple to silver and eventually they'll look like pale streaks on your skin.

Shrinking piles (haemorrhoids)

You may have developed piles during your pregnancy. Piles are swollen blood vessels in or around the anus and lower rectum. They are very common during pregnancy because carrying your baby in the womb and childbirth itself put pressure on the blood vessels and affect blood circulation. Also, the pregnancy hormone progesterone relaxes the blood vessels and slows down blood flow, making the veins swell. If you suffered from constipation during your pregnancy this would have also increased the pressure on the veins.

Your piles should gradually shrink without any treatment as your body and circulation returns to normal. To help the process along eat plenty of fibre-rich foods, such as wholegrain bread, brown rice, fruit, vegetables and beans, and drink plenty of fluids. If the piles feel sore or itchy apply an over-the-counter haemorrhoid cream, which will shrink them and soothe the soreness and irritation. If you find sitting down uncomfortable you could try using an inflatable cushion (see page 175). If they continue to cause you problems a few weeks after the birth tell your GP.

Thinner hair

During pregnancy, the extra oestrogen extends your hair's growth cycle, so you lose less hair than usual. This is why many women notice their hair is thicker while they are pregnant. After the birth, as your oestrogen levels return to normal, you will probably notice that you are losing more hair than usual; don't worry – you won't go bald! This is just a sign that your hair is returning to its normal growth cycle – which can take a few months.

> ### Postnatal check-up
>
> You'll be offered a postnatal check-up with your GP around six weeks after the birth. Your doctor should discuss how you are feeling physically and emotionally, to make sure you're recovering well[20]. However, you can contact your GP at any stage if you have any concerns about yourself or your baby.

As well as changes to your body you will also probably notice changes in your emotions.

Be prepared for the baby blues

It's normal for new mums to feel a little weepy and emotional a few days after the birth. This is thought to be due to the sudden drop in hormone levels after giving birth. Also, you have just been through a life-changing event – your life will never be the same again and you are coping with the demands of caring for a tiny human being who is totally reliant on you for their every need. Add to that the fact that your sleep is being disturbed each night and it's easy to understand why you might feel a little low. Baby blues symptoms include feeling weepy and upset, often for no obvious reason. It usually only lasts for a few days and often just being aware that this is normal and perhaps talking to another mother or confiding in your partner, a relative or friend about your feelings will be enough to help you cope. However it is important not to mistake the baby blues for postnatal illness (PNI), previously known as postnatal depression (PND), which is a much more severe condition and affects around one in seven mothers. Up to one in ten dads/partners are thought to suffer from depression after the birth of their baby too.

Recognise postnatal illness (PNI)

If you continue to feel low, feel worse, or begin feeling very low at any time in the first year you could be suffering from postnatal illness. The symptoms to watch out for in yourself and your partner include:

▶ Tearfulness, crying

▶ Feeling anxious

▶ Panic attacks

▶ Feeling isolated

▶ Difficulty sleeping

▶ Feeling exhausted – even after sleep

▶ Suffering from nightmares

▶ Suffering from flashbacks of your labour and birth

▶ Physical symptoms like chest pain, headaches, feeling dizzy

▶ Worrying obsessively about your or your baby's health

▶ Worrying obsessively about cot death

▶ Worrying about harming your baby

▶ Feeling that you can't look after your baby properly

- ▶ Failure to bond with your baby

- ▶ Feeling overwhelmed

- ▶ Lacking emotion

- ▶ Self-harming

- ▶ Suicidal thoughts and feelings

Be aware of the risk factors for PNI

While hormones may be a factor, it is thought that the huge changes that becoming a parent brings, such as the extra responsibilities, financial pressures and lack of sleep are also involved. This is borne out by the fact that partners can also suffer from the condition. Research suggests that depression can be 'catching', so if one parent is feeling depressed the other one is likely to be affected too. Other risk factors include:

- ▶ Previous history of depression

- ▶ Lack of support from your partner/family

- ▶ Having a premature or poorly baby

- ▶ Recent stressful event such as bereavement or a house move

However, it is possible to develop PNI for no obvious reason.

What to do if you think you or your partner have PNI

If you think you or your partner may be suffering from PNI it is vital that you tell your midwife, health visitor or GP as soon as you can. They will assess the severity of your depression and offer you appropriate treatment. For mild depression they may just monitor you and suggest ways you can help yourself – such as arranging a babysitter so you can have a night off. For moderate depression they may suggest counselling, such as cognitive behavioural therapy (CBT). CBT aims to help you change the way you feel and act by teaching you how to challenge any negative thoughts you have about yourself and your life and replace them with more positive ones. There is usually a long waiting list for this treatment, but there are online courses you can access through the NHS, if your GP refers you and your local clinical commissioning group is willing to fund one. These include:

Beating the Blues – this course consists of eight 50-minute sessions for people with depression and anxiety. The programme aims to teach you strategies you can use to help you cope better with day-to-day life.

FearFighter – this is a ten-week course for people suffering from anxiety or a phobia. The course aims to teach you how to face your fears and lead a normal life, and can be completed at your own pace.

If your GP is unable to refer you onto one of these CBT courses there are others that are available free of charge such as:

MoodGYM – an online programme that teaches cognitive behavioural therapy skills to help you prevent and deal with depression.

E-couch – a self-help interactive programme with modules on topics like depression, anxiety, relationship breakdown, and loss and grief. It teaches you how to use strategies from cognitive, behavioural and interpersonal therapies, as well as relaxation and physical activity.

Living Life to the Full – an online life-skills course that uses CBT techniques to help you overcome anxiety and depression.

For further information on all of these courses see the Directory, page 198.

> PNI ORG UK is a charity set up by PNI sufferers for PNI sufferers. It offers support via a forum, which can help you cope with the illness – from getting help, through your recovery and beyond. For details of this organisation and others that exist to help parents with PNI see the Directory, page 198.

Ask for help

Asking your partner and family for more help and support – perhaps by taking over some of the household chores or by babysitting once a week, so that you can have some 'me time' – could help to ease the pressure. You might use that 'me time' to do something as simple as indulging in a long hot soak in the bath, or reading a book, or you might want to get out of the house for a bit of pampering like getting your hair done or having an aromatherapy massage.

Look after yourself

Eating well, taking gentle exercise, resting when you can, managing your stress levels and generally being kind to yourself will help with your recovery and can help prevent PNI from developing in the first place. It isn't selfish to think of your own needs – it is vitally important for your emotional and physical well-being. Remember you won't be able to look after your baby to the best of your ability if you are feeling unhappy or unwell.

Eat well

Whether or not you are breastfeeding, now is not the time to go on a strict diet. Instead aim to eat sensibly.

Try to avoid relying on ready meals – ask your partner if they could cook for the first few weeks – or at least until you have recovered from the birth and established some kind of routine. If you have time before the birth you could cook some healthy meals and freeze them so that you have a supply of ready prepared meals when you need them. When you do start cooking choose uncomplicated recipes that can be prepared quickly.

Make sure you eat a source of good quality protein at every meal – for example eggs, fish, chicken or lean meat; these will keep you feeling full for longer and provide important amino acids that are essential for cell growth and repair. Eating oily fish such as sardines, salmon, mackerel or fresh tuna a couple of times a week will help to ensure that you get enough omega-3 fatty acids. A handful of nuts or seeds will supply magnesium and omega-6 fatty acids. Your baby needs omega-3 and omega-6 fatty acids for healthy brain development, so if you are breastfeeding it is especially important that you get enough of these nutrients. Include dairy foods such as milk, yoghurt and cheese to ensure you get enough calcium. Full-fat products are now considered healthier than low-fat versions, which tend to contain extra sugar and other additives. Also, full-fat dairy foods keep you feeling full for longer, so you are less likely to want to snack between meals.

Whole grains – such as wholemeal bread, porridge oats, brown rice, pulses and whole-wheat pasta will provide slow-release energy to keep your blood sugar steady so that you feel full for longer and are less likely to want to snack on biscuits, cakes and sweets, which supply plentiful calories with few nutrients. However, recent research suggests that eating too many carbohydrate-rich foods can lead to weight gain; so if you are trying to lose the baby-weight you might want to limit your intake of these foods to no more than six portions a day. As a rough guide a portion is equal to one slice of bread, three tablespoons of cooked pasta, two tablespoons of cooked rice, two small boiled potatoes or half a baked potato. Eat plenty of fruit and vegetables for fibre, antioxidants, vitamins and minerals. This type of diet will supply you (and your baby if you're breastfeeding) with all the nutrients you need for good health. Breastfeeding mums in particular should not attempt to diet, but aim to eat sensibly.

Drink plenty of fluids – but curb the caffeine

Make sure you drink plenty of fluids – this can include tea and coffee, but avoid drinking more than three or four mugs daily as the caffeine can cause insomnia and anxiety. It's hard to say how much caffeine is too much, as some people are more sensitive to it than others – but experts suggest limiting your intake to no more than 300 mg a day; this is especially important if you are breastfeeding, as caffeine passes into your milk and your baby's liver breaks down caffeine much more slowly than yours does. Remember cola, cocoa and chocolate also contain caffeine. The amount of caffeine in a drink varies according to the size of the cup, the amount of tea or coffee used and the time it is left to brew. Try replacing caffeinated drinks with decaffeinated teas and coffees and caffeine-free herbal teas, such as peppermint, chamomile, lemon and ginger and Redbush. Bear in mind though that green tea contains around 25 mg of caffeine. If you are breastfeeding you don't need to drink excessive amounts of liquid, but make sure you drink whenever you feel thirsty – no matter how busy you are and have a glass of water to hand when feeding.

Caffeine in tea, coffee, cocoa and chocolate

Drink/Food	Caffeine Content
Tea (mug)	55–140 mg
Instant coffee (cup)	54 mg (on average)
Ground coffee (cup)	105 mg (on average)
Cocoa (cup)	5 mg (on average)
50 g plain chocolate	Up to 50 mg
50 g milk chocolate	25 mg (on average)

Watch your alcohol intake

While a glass of wine will help you to relax, avoid drinking more than one a day. If you drink more than that your ability to look after your baby might be impaired. Also, if you like to co-sleep with your baby there is the danger that you could sleep so soundly that you roll onto your baby without realising, or forget your baby is there and roll onto them.

If you are suffering from PNI don't be tempted to drink to make you feel better – alcohol depletes vitamin B1 and magnesium from the body; both of these nutrients are needed for a healthy nervous system, so a lack of them could make your depression worse.

If you are breastfeeding it's important to be aware that alcohol will go into your breast milk about 30 minutes after you have a drink. The level of alcohol in your breast milk will be more or less the same as the level in your bloodstream. Your blood-alcohol level will be highest between 30 and 60 minutes after you have a drink, or 90 minutes if you have a drink with a meal. It takes around one hour for one unit of alcohol to leave your blood (the smaller you are the longer it will take); so if you intend to have a drink aim to have one straight after a feed, so that your body can process it before the next one. One unit is roughly equal to one small (125 ml) glass of wine, half a pint of beer or lager (depending on the strength) one small glass of sherry or port or one single measure of spirits.

Regular heavy drinking could affect your baby's development. Also, research suggests that alcohol can hamper the letdown of your milk and babies take less milk from their mother after she has had a drink – possibly because it tastes different. So it is advisable to drink no more than one or two units once or twice a week when you are breastfeeding. If you plan to drink more than this for a special occasion, it is a good idea to express some milk beforehand so that your baby can have an alcohol-free feed.

Take regular gentle exercise

Pregnancy and childbirth are the biggest challenges a woman's body will ever face, so don't expect to return to your normal shape and fitness straight away; it should be a gradual process. Listen to your body and don't overdo things – especially in the early days and if you are establishing breastfeeding. Aim to do 30 minutes of gentle exercise a day – such as taking your baby for a walk in the pram buggy, or sling. Walking is relatively easy to fit in to a busy day, even if it is just a walk around the supermarket or to the park. While it is a gentle form of exercise, it not only burns calories and aids weight loss but also offers a host of other health benefits including improved cardiovascular fitness, lower blood pressure, stronger bones and muscles and improved mood. Pushing the pram or carrying your baby will help to improve your muscle tone and burn extra calories.

If you can't get outdoors, just doing light housework and going up and down stairs will give you the opportunity to be active. As you regain your strength and get settled into a breastfeeding routine you will find that you can gradually increase the amount of time you are active each day. Don't attempt strenuous exercise until you have been given the all-clear from your doctor. This is usually at your six-week check-up if you had a normal delivery or at eight weeks if you had a Caesarean section.

> **Tighten your pelvic floor and tummy**
>
> You can help your pelvic floor return to normal after having your baby by stopping your urine mid flow and holding for a few seconds. Tone your tummy by taking a deep breath in to a count of five, holding for 5 seconds and then pulling your tummy in as you breathe out to a count of five. Repeat up to ten times every day.

Deal with stress

Coping with a crying baby and lack of sleep as well as getting to grips with new skills like feeding and caring for your baby can leave you feeling under a lot of pressure. Taking a few minutes to de-stress every day can help you feel calmer. Here are a few stress-relieving techniques to help you redress the balance when you are feeling overwhelmed.

Instant calm meditation

If you are feeling frazzled, calm down with this mindfulness meditation that only takes a couple of minutes.

1. Sit down and choose an object in the room, or something you can see through your window. It could be your coffee table or a tree outside.

2. Breathe in slowly and deeply through your nose to a count of five. Hold for a count of five then exhale slowly through your mouth to a count of five.

3. Continue to inhale, hold your breath and exhale at roughly the same pace. At the same time focus on your chosen object and notice every detail – for example the colour, size and shape of the coffee table, or the colour and texture of the leaves and the bark on the tree. Do this for a minute or two whenever the stresses of parenthood are getting to you and you should feel instantly calmer.

Challenge your negative thoughts

According to CBT your feelings aren't facts – they are just your perception of an event or situation. In other words, an event or situation is only stressful if you think it is. How you view and respond to situations is down to the filters you view them through. These filters include your personality, values, beliefs and attitudes, which are the result of your genetics, upbringing, past experiences, lifestyle and culture. However, it is possible to change how you view a situation and your reaction to it, simply by changing your beliefs about yourself and situations. Below is an example of how you can use CBT to help you cope with the stresses of parenthood.

Situation: Your baby cries a lot every evening.

Negative thought: I must be doing something wrong.

Consequences of negative thought: Feeling stressed and unable to cope.

Challenge your negative thought: By viewing the situation differently, for example: 'Lots of babies cry, it doesn't mean I'm doing anything wrong, maybe my baby has colic.' This can make you feel more positive and act accordingly.

Response to new way of thinking: I'll find out more about colic and how to deal with it.

Result of new approach: Feeling more positive and in control.

Get outdoors

Research shows that getting outdoors into a 'green space', such as a garden, park or woodland cuts stress levels, lifts our mood and makes us feel more relaxed and confident. Just stopping and admiring a pleasant view has been shown to lower the amount of the stress hormone cortisol in the blood by 13 per cent. The Japanese call the grounding, calming effect of looking at trees *shinrin-yoku*, which means 'forest bathing'. Walking encourages the body to release the 'happy hormone' serotonin and naturally tranquilising endorphins. Also, getting outside in daylight will help both you and your baby sleep better at night, because it encourages the body to produce the sleep hormone melatonin at night. So when you're feeling stressed why not get yourself and your baby ready and head off outdoors?

Have fun with your baby

It's all too easy to feel bogged down with the practicalities of looking after your baby and running your home and forget to have fun and enjoy being with them. Playing peek-a-boo with your baby, or giving them a soothing massage (see page 115) – will help you relax and seeing them smile will lift your mood.

Real-life tips on surviving early parenthood

Amber, 33 – first-time mum to Jack

'For me the first two weeks were very scary. I felt out of my depth. My husband and I worried a lot. Was Jack too cold or too hot? Was he getting enough milk? I cried a lot. It took me till about 2 p.m. each day to get ready to go out – even with my husband's help!

'My advice to new mums would be to get a routine as fast as you can. Once I had a routine I found it made life easier.'

Sam, 32 – first-time mum to Holly

'Don't expect to be "supermum" after the birth, because it isn't going to happen. Take it easy or you'll struggle to recover. I did too much too quickly and the next day paid the price. I felt dreadful and the postpartum bleeding doubled, which I read was your body telling you to slow down and it was probably right.

'Be strict with visitors and make sure you have time as a family to get used to having a baby and enjoy those first few weeks. All the books tell you to plan food in advance and freeze it down – I didn't, but it would have been helpful.

'Try to be as prepared as possible – have everything you can in for the baby, so you don't have to go out shopping, etc.'

Chris 33 – first-time dad to Holly

'In the weeks after the birth I supported Sam by doing housework and cooking, walking the dog, changing nappies and helping to bath Holly. I also gave Sam my verbal support by telling her how good she was with the baby. I think that helped to boost her confidence in the early days. I started to relax more as a parent once I realised that when my baby cried she just wanted simple things like food, sleep, or a nappy change.'

And finally...

This book has offered you lots of advice on how to care for your new baby and cope with the physical and emotional changes that childbirth brings. The final sections of the book offer you details of products you may find useful and a list of books you may find helpful if you want to learn more about some of the topics covered in the book. You'll also find contact details, including web addresses of organisations that you may want to consult for further information and support. I hope this guide has addressed many of your questions and concerns about becoming a parent for the first time and has helped you along your parenting journey.

HELPFUL FURTHER READING

Hogg, Tracy and Blau, Melinda, *Secrets Of The Baby Whisperer: How to Calm, Connect and Communicate with your Baby* (Vermilion, 2001) – a useful guide to help you understand yourself and your baby and work out what kind of parenting suits you both.

La Leche League International, *The Womanly Art of Breastfeeding* (Pinter & Martin Ltd., 2010) – an invaluable guide to establishing and maintaining breastfeeding.

Modell, Stephanie, *The Baby Sleep Guide: Practical Advice to Establish Good Sleep Habits* (Summersdale, 2015) – this book contains a wealth of information on how to encourage your baby to develop good sleep habits from early on.

First Aid for Babies and Children Fast (Dorling Kindersley, 2012) – written in association with the British Red Cross, this guide explains how to treat over 100 conditions that could affect your baby/child.

USEFUL PRODUCTS

Below is a list of baby products and suppliers of baby products that you may find useful in the first three months of being a parent. The author doesn't endorse nor recommend any particular product and this list is by no means exhaustive.

Angelcare sound and movement monitor

An under-the-mattress sensor pad that monitors your baby's movements; if your baby is still for 20 seconds an alarm goes off to alert you.

Website: www.angelcareuk.co.uk

Aveeno bath and shower oil

A bath oil containing natural oils, vitamin E and oatmeal to soothe dry, eczema prone skin. Suitable for babies from three months.

Website: www.aveeno.co.uk

Babasling

A one-size 100 per cent cotton adjustable sling designed to carry babies and toddlers weighing 7 lb 11oz to 33 lb 1 oz (3.5–15 kg). It has five different carrying positions, including two that allow you to breastfeed discreetly. Has a lifetime guarantee against manufacturing defects.

Website: www.thebabasling.com

Balneum Medicinal Bath Oil

Treats dry skin associated with eczema. Suitable for babies. Available over-the-counter at pharmacies.

Website: www.almirall.com

BioGaia ProTectis

Probiotic baby drops containing *Lactobacillus reuteri* to treat wind and colic. May also help to prevent gastroenteritis in bottle-fed babies.

Website: www.biogaia.co.uk

Breastvest

A vest designed to enable breastfeeding mums to feed more discreetly in public. It comes to below the breast and you wear a normal top over it. When you want to feed your baby you lift your top and bra and your tummy stays covered.

Website: www.breastvest.co.uk

Calpol Soothe & Care Saline Nasal Spray/ Saline Drops

Help to wash away built up mucus from your baby's nose. Suitable to use from birth.

Website: www.calpol.co.uk

Cussons Mum & Me Sleep Tight Massage Oil

Reasonably priced hypoallergenic baby massage oil containing grape seed, peach kernel, jojoba, jasmine and aloe vera leaf extracts.

Website: www.mumandme.com

Earth Mama Angel Baby Organic Milkmaid Tea

Herbal tea that may help to boost milk production in breastfeeding mothers. Ingredients include fennel, fenugreek and caraway seeds, raspberry leaf, nettle leaf and milk thistle.

Website: www.expressyourselfmums.co.uk

Feed-Finder

Feed-finder is an app you can use to find breastfeeding-friendly venues when you are out and about.

Website: www.feed-finder.co.uk

Lansinoh HPA Lanolin Nipple Cream

Lansinoh is a hypoallergenic lanolin cream to help heal and protect sore, cracked nipples in breastfeeding mothers. It is available over the counter in most pharmacies.

Website: www.lansinoh.co.uk

Oilatum Junior

A range of fragrance-free skin care products for babies and children with dry, eczema-prone skin. The range includes a lotion, cream and bath additive that contain moisturisers and mineral oils to support the skin's natural barrier.

Website: www.oilatum.co.uk

Snufflebabe Nasal Aspirator

Paediatrician-approved aspirator to clear babies' blocked noses. Safe to use from birth.

Website: www.snufflebabe.co.uk

Snufflebabe Vapour Oil

Vapour oil containing lemon, pine and tea tree essential oils. Safe for use from birth in your baby's room and can be added to a bowl of warm water, or with some vaporisers and humidifiers.

Website: www.snufflebabe.co.uk

VALLEY Cushion

An inflatable cushion designed to ease discomfort when sitting after procedures like an episiotomy or conditions like haemorrhoids (piles).

Website: www.valleycushions.co.uk

DIRECTORY

Association of Breastfeeding Mothers

Offers breastfeeding counselling via the telephone, letter and email. The website offers up-to-date breastfeeding information and details of their breastfeeding support groups in the UK.

Address: ABM, PO Box 207, Bridgwater, Somerset TA6 7YT
Helpline: 0300 330 5453
Email: online contact form
Website: abm.me.uk

The Association for Post-Natal Illness

Offers support to mothers suffering from postnatal illness (PNI) and aims to raise public awareness of the illness. Provides information, a telephone helpline and a network of volunteers who have experienced postnatal illness.

Address: 145 Dawes Road, Fulham, London SW6 7EB
Helpline: 0171 386 0868
Website: www.apni.org

The Baby Café

Part of the National Childbirth Trust (NCT) charity. It coordinates a network of breastfeeding drop-in centres and other services to support breastfeeding mothers across the UK and other parts of the world.

Address: The Baby Café, Alexandra House, Oldham Terrace, London W3 6NH

Email: online contact form
Website: www.thebabycafe.org

Baby Centre UK

Website for new and expectant parents offering information on a wide range of topics, such as breastfeeding, or choosing a name for your baby.

Website: www.babycentre.co.uk

Beating the Blues

A cognitive behavioural therapy (CBT) based course made up of eight online sessions to treat people who are stressed, depressed or anxious. If your GP diagnoses you with depression, they can refer you for the course via the NHS.

Website: www.beatingtheblues.co.uk

The Breastfeeding Network

A Scottish charity that offers information, live online chat support, telephone support and drop-in centres for breastfeeding mothers across the UK.

Address: The Breastfeeding Network, PO Box 11126, Paisley PA2 8YB
Telephone: BfN Supporter line: 0300 100 0210
Helpline: 0300 100 0212
Email: Admin@breastfeedingnetwork.org.uk
Website: www.breastfeedingnetwork.org.uk

Breastfeeding Welcome Scheme

A scheme run by the National Childbirth Trust to help breastfeeding women identify venues that welcome breastfeeding mothers. There is a venue locator on the website to enable you to find breastfeeding friendly venues wherever you are.

Address: Alexandra House, Oldham Terrace, London, W3 6NH
Email: online contact form
Website: www.breastfeedingwelcomescheme.org.uk

Cry-sis

A UK charity offering information and emotional support to families with excessively crying, sleepless and demanding babies; they also offer a helpline with trained volunteers.

Address: BM Cry-sis, London WC1N 3XX
Helpline: 08451 228 669 (all year daily 9 a.m.–10 p.m.)
Website: www.cry-sis.org.uk

E-couch

A self-help interactive programme with modules on topics like depression, anxiety, relationship breakdown, and loss and grief. It teaches you how to use strategies from cognitive, behavioural and interpersonal therapies, as well as relaxation techniques and physical activity.

Website: www.ecouch.anu.edu.au

Family Lives

A UK charity providing a range of national and local services, including a confidential helpline to support parents and families across the country, before they reach crisis point. Address: Family Lives Head Office, 49–51 East Road, London N1 6AH

Helpline: 0808 800 2222
Email: online contact form
Website: www.familylives.org.uk

Fearfighter

An online programme that uses CBT to help tackle anxiety and is available on the NHS where local CCGs have commissioned it, or you can buy it privately online.

Website: www.fearfighter.com

Gentle Parenting

A website that aims to provide evidence-based information for parents that is always in the best interest of the child, as well as greater society.

Website: www.gentleparenting.co.uk

Gurgle

A parenting website, linked to the magazine of the same name. It offers useful guides on various topics including pregnancy, caring for your newborn and breastfeeding.

Website: www.gurgle.com

Home Start

Offers one-to-one support to help families cope with babies and young children in the form of a volunteer who visits the family's home for a couple of hours every week. They also run family groups and social events for families.

Helpline: 08000 68 63 68 (Mon–Fri 8 a.m.–8 p.m. and Sat 9 a.m.–noon)
Website: www.home-start.org.uk

International Association of Infant Massage

Offers baby massage instructor training and baby massage classes across the UK.

Address: IAIM UK Chapter, Unit 10 Marlborough Business Centre, 96 George Lane, South Woodford, London E18 1AD
Telephone: 020 8989 9597
Email: online contact form
Website: www.iaim.org.uk

La Leche League

A registered charity that aims to help mothers worldwide to breastfeed through mother-to-mother support, encouragement, information, and education, and to promote a better understanding of breastfeeding. The website offers information and forums.

Helpline: 0845 120 2918
Email: online contact forms to contact your local group or to submit a request for help
Website: www.laleche.org.uk

Living Life to the Full

An online life-skills course that uses CBT techniques to help you overcome anxiety and depression.

Website: www.llttf.com

Lullaby Trust

Provides information on preventing sudden infant death syndrome (SIDS) and specialist support for bereaved families and anyone affected by a SID.

Address: 11 Belgrave Road, London SW1V 1RB
General enquiries: 020 7802 3200 **Information line:** 0808 802 6869
Bereavement support: 0808 802 6868

Email: office@lullabytrust.org.uk
Website: www.lullabytrust.org.uk

Made for Mums

Made For Mums is a website run by a small group of journalists, offering information, online discussions and news on all aspects of childcare right through from pregnancy, to caring for a baby, toddler and school-age children.

Address: Made For Mums, Immediate Media Co., Vineyard House, 44 Brook Green, Hammersmith. London W6 7BT
Email: contactus@madeformums.com
Website: www. madeformums.com

MoodGYM

An online programme that teaches cognitive behavioural therapy skills (CBT) to help prevent and deal with depression.

Website: http://moodgym.anu.edu.au

Mumsnet

An online community for parents. The website's aim is to make parents' lives easier by pooling knowledge, experience and support.

Website: www.mumsnet.com

National Childbirth Trust

A UK charity offering information and support during pregnancy, birth, and early parenthood. The charity has a nationwide network of local branches to reach and support all parents and parents-to-be, as well as courses and telephone helplines.

Address: Alexandra House, Oldham Terrace, London W3 6NH
Helpline: 0300 330 0700
Email: complete online contact form
Website: www.nct.org.uk

Netmums

Netmums is a local network that offers information and advice on being a mum including a directory of services in your local area. The website offers information on a range of topics including feeding your baby, baby health and baby sleep.

Website: www.netmums.com

PNI ORG UK

A website and forum run by sufferers and past sufferers of postnatal illness (PNI) offering information and one-to-one-support via the forum and email.

Email: one2onesupport@pni.org.uk
Website: www.pni.org.uk

Sure Start

Sure Start is a government initiative to support parents from pregnancy and give young children from the most disadvantaged areas the best possible start in life. Sure Start Children's Centres offer postnatal support such as breastfeeding support programmes, baby massage, baby yoga and play sessions.

Telephone: 0370 000 2288
Website: www.nidirect.gov.uk/sure-start-services

REFERENCES

1 NHS Choices 2013, 2014

2 Heller et al 2012

3 Unicef 2011

4 NHS Choices 2012

5 Crawley and Westland 2013

6 FSA/NHS 2012

7 FSA/NHS 2012

8 FSA/NHS 2012

9 Crawley and Westland 2013

10 Crawley and Westland 2013, NHS 2012b

11 NHS 2012c, UNICEF 2012

12 NHS 2013a

13 AWHONN 2013, NHS Choices 2013

14 NHS Scotland 2007

15 Ficca et al 2000, Davis et al 2004

16 DH 2009: 120

17 NICE 2009: 1, NHS 2011a, Tidy 2010

18 NHS 2010d

19 CKS 2009, NHS 2011

20 DH 2009a, NICE 2006

THE
BABY SLEEP
GUIDE

Practical Advice to
Establish Good Sleep Habits

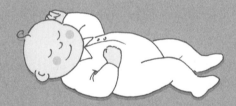

- Establish good bedtime and nap routines
- Understand how your baby sleeps
- Help your baby to self-settle
- Learn about sleep cycles

From Birth to 1 Year

Stephanie Modell
Foreword by Jill Irving
RN (adult) RN (child) RM RHV JP

THE BABY SLEEP GUIDE

Practical Advice to Establish Good Sleep Habits

Stephanie Modell

£6.99
Paperback
ISBN: 978-1-84953-685-1

Babies do wake at night, but you can help them learn to sleep with some gentle guidance.

Sleep. It's the most precious commodity, especially when you're struggling to find it. The secret to helping your baby to sleep through is understanding their sleep cycles and natural rhythms. *The Baby Sleep Guide* provides simple and easy techniques to help you establish positive sleep habits early on that will pay dividends in the long term. It guides you through different sleep teaching approaches so you can find a healthy balance that works for you and your baby. Designed to be deliberately concise to find information at a glance, *The Baby Sleep Guide* offers clear solutions to ensure a good night's sleep for everyone.

Have you enjoyed this book?
If so, why not write a review on your favourite website?

If you're interested in finding out more about our books,
find us on Facebook at **Summersdale Publishers** and
follow us on Twitter at **@Summersdale**.

Thanks very much for buying this Summersdale book.

www.summersdale.com